PANDEMIC SPOTLIGHT

PANDEMIC SPOTLIGHT

Canadian Doctors at the Front of the COVID-19 Fight

Ian Hanomansing

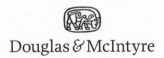

Douglas & McIntyre

DOUGLAS AND MCINTYRE (2013) LTD.
P.O. Box 219, Madeira Park, BC, V0N 2H0
www.douglas-mcintyre.com

Edited and indexed by Audrey McClellan
Cover and text design by Shed Simas / Onça Design
Printed and bound in Canada
100% recycled paper content

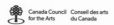 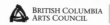

Douglas and McIntyre acknowledges the support of the Canada Council for the Arts, the Government of Canada, and the Province of British Columbia through the BC Arts Council.

LIBRARY AND ARCHIVES CANADA CATALOGUING IN PUBLICATION
Title: Pandemic spotlight : Canadian doctors at the front of the COVID-19 fight / Ian Hanomansing.
Names: Hanomansing, Ian, author.
Description: Includes index.
Identifiers: Canadiana (print) 20210272783 | Canadiana (ebook) 20210272805 | ISBN 9781771622929 (softcover) | ISBN 9781771622936 (EPUB)
Subjects: LCSH: COVID-19 Pandemic, 2020-—Canada. | LCSH: Medical personnel—Canada. | LCSH: Communication in public health—Canada.
Classification: LCC RA644.C67 H36 2021 | DDC 362.1962/41400971—dc23

To the many victims of the pandemic: those who died, those whose illnesses were life changing. To their families and the health care workers who cared for them.

And, on a personal note, to my parents, Harvey and Eunice, and my sister, Ria.

And to my wife, Nancy, and our sons, Daniel and James.

I've been fortunate to live in two households that treasure words, ideas and debate.

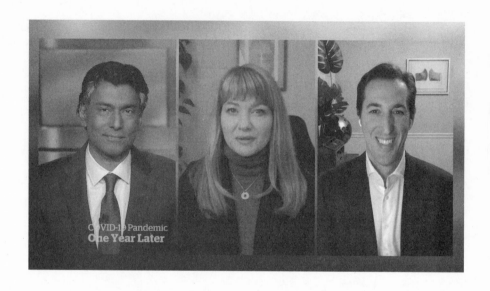

Ian Hanomansing speaks to doctors Lynora Saxinger and Isaac Bogoch on CBC News: *The National.*
Photo courtesy CBC

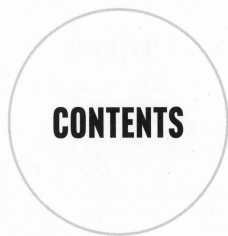

CONTENTS

TIMELINE

2019

December 30   ProMed alert sent to doctors about a pneumonia of "unknown origin" in Wuhan, China

2020

January 25   First "presumptive" case found in Canada

February 11   World Health Organization (WHO) announces name of this new respiratory disease—COVID-19

February 20   BC announces first case not connected to travel in China

March 8   First confirmed Canadian death due to Covid

March 11   WHO declares a pandemic

March 17   Ontario Premier Doug Ford declares a state of emergency, closing indoor recreation facilities, restaurants, libraries, theatres and concert halls. Other provinces follow suit. In BC, in-person classes are cancelled indefinitely

March 20   US/Canada border is closed to all non-essential travel

March 25   Atlantic provinces prohibit "unnecessary travel" from other provinces

May 20   Chief Public Health Officer of Canada Theresa Tam recommends Canadians wear non-medical masks

June 24   As cases flatten, BC moves to phase 3 allowing responsible travel and tourism

July 3   "Atlantic Bubble" allows residents of the four eastern provinces to travel within Atlantic Canada

November 26   "Atlantic Bubble" suspended due to rising Covid cases during the second wave

December 9	Health Canada approves first vaccine for COVID-19, the Pfizer BioNTech vaccine and vaccinations soon begin across Canada, prioritizing long-term care homes
December 26	Ontario implements "Provincewide Lockdown" for 28 days because of concerns over rising hospitalizations

2021

January 4	Diagnoses of new COVID-19 cases peak in Canada, with over 14,000 new cases in a single day
January 9	Quebec imposes curfew to restrict gatherings in evenings. Originally announced as a 28-day measure, it is in place for 139 days
January 13	COVID-19 hospitalizations in Canada peak, with 4,868 patients reported in hospitals
January 14	Ontario moves to stricter "Stay at Home Order"
March 30	BC announces "circuit breaker" with new restrictions on in-person interactions
April 6	Concerns over third wave prompt Alberta government to introduce stricter measures
April 13	Citing apprehension over sharp rise in "variants of concern" the government of Saskatchewan brings in tighter restrictions, including limiting "household bubbles" to immediate households only
April 23	BC prohibits non-essential travel within the province
May 25	As the third wave diminishes, BC implements first of four stage "Restart" plan, to lift Covid restrictions over four months
May 28	Quebec lifts curfew and eases other restrictions
July 1	Many Canadian provinces, including Alberta, BC and Nova Scotia, ease COVID-19 restrictions, including mandatory mask regulations
July 30	81% of Canadians aged 12 and older have received at least one COVID-19 vaccination; 68% are fully vaccinated. Most universities, schools and workplaces plan to re-open fully by fall

SELECT ABBREVIATIONS

DTM&H	Diploma in Tropical Medicine and Hygiene
FRCPC	Fellow of the Royal College of Physicians of Canada
H1N1	a subtype of the Influenza A virus, which can cause influenza in humans
ICU	intensive care unit
ID	infectious diseases
MIS-C	multi system inflammatory syndrome in children
mRNA	messenger RNA—Pfizer and Moderna are mRNA vaccines
NACI	National Advisory Council on Immunization
NIH	National Institutes of Health
NIAD	National Institute of Allergy and Infectious Disease
PPE	personal protective equipment
ProMED	Program for Monitoring Emerging Diseases
SARS	severe acute respiratory syndrome
SARS-CoV-2	severe acute respiratory syndrome coronavirus 2, the virus that causes COVID-19
VITT	vaccine-induced immune thrombotic thrombocytopenia, rare blood clots associated with the AstraZeneca vaccine

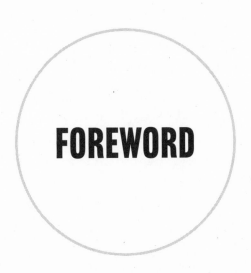

FOREWORD

ONE OF THE INTRIGUING THINGS ABOUT WRITING A BOOK is imagining who's reading it. Perhaps you're a CBC viewer or listener, eager to find out more about the infectious disease doctors who have become so familiar to Canadians. But it's also possible you picked this up at a yard sale, years after it was published, curious about the Great Pandemic of 2020–21.

In that case, let me tell you a little about myself and how this book came to be. I've been a journalist for a long time. As I write this, in Vancouver in June 2021, I have two main assignments: anchoring *The National*, CBC TV's nightly newscast, on Fridays and Sundays; and filling in for the last few months as host of *Cross Country Checkup*, a weekly national call-in show on CBC Radio.

Over the years I've had the privilege to witness many historic moments. My first major assignment came when I was twenty-seven years old, in March 1989. My colleagues and I jumped on a plane to head to Valdez, Alaska, to cover the massive oil spill that occurred when the *Exxon Valdez* hit a reef. Since then I have reported on many more big stories, in the field and from the desk. Riots and elections. Notorious murders and tragic plane crashes. On June 30, 1997, I woke up in the British colony of Hong Kong, and when I returned to my hotel in the early hours of July 1, I was in China's new Special Administrative Region.

Urgent at the time, most of these headline stories diminish in impact surprisingly quickly. But over my more than three decades of reporting, there have been two notable exceptions. The first is 9/11. I was in Vancouver when the planes hit the World Trade Center towers, and I was sent to the Canada–US border, about a thirty-minute drive south of the city. For the first time, it was closed. Not just to non-essential travellers but shut completely. Reporters, travellers and border guards walked around, speaking in hushed, shocked tones about what had happened on the other side of the continent.

For days, every minute of every newscast was devoted to the attack. We even did a story a couple of weeks later about the other stories that we hadn't had room for. I never imagined there would be something that could dominate even more of our coverage. That is, until the spring of 2020.

One of the most overused words of the pandemic has been "unprecedented," but it does describe how Covid affected the news. Every story on every day for weeks was connected to this new, frightening virus. The number of people watching, reading and listening to the news surged. We were all so desperate for information. Much of that came from government leaders and health officials. But, as always, we in the media needed more. We needed explanations and, perhaps above all, reassurance. What should we do to try to stay safe?

Stepping into the void, one by one, across the country, was a group of infectious disease doctors. It was a remarkable thing to see. Experts being interviewed in the media is not, by itself, unusual. On every one of those big headline stories I mentioned earlier, we would go to academics or lawyers or former police officers or pilots who would, for a day or at most a week, help us understand what was going on.

But the pandemic wasn't just a week or a month or even a year. And yet, these doctors kept coming back, never paid for their time and expertise, never making us feel like we were imposing. The more I interviewed them on *The National* and *Cross Country Checkup*, the more I was not just impressed, but also increasingly curious. However, like many of you, I knew virtually nothing about them, until I wrote this book.

Even as I write that phrase—"wrote this book"—it seems strange and exciting. I've written a lot of words over the years, but only to be read by me, a few seconds at a time, on TV or radio. I did consider profiling these doctors in a news story or maybe a podcast. But in the end their stories deserved the detail and permanence of a book.

I sent each of them an email back in February 2021, wondering if they'd be willing to spend a couple of hours on the phone and speak candidly about their lives before and during the pandemic. I watched my inbox anxiously, and within hours, one by one, they all said yes.

One last thing: the doctors volunteered their time—a lot of time—to those of us in the media. In keeping with that, I am volunteering my time in writing this book. All royalties are being donated to the University of British Columbia medical school. More specifically, to the Future of Public Health Fund at the UBC School of Population and Public Health. The Faculty of Medicine describes the donation this way: *This fund provides a great opportunity to support students studying infectious diseases or public health at UBC. As the backbone of the province's home-grown expertise in public health, the School works tirelessly to promote health and well-being for everyone. Thus, your gift would contribute to a large-scale, equitable and meaningful impact.*

I hope you enjoy this book a little more, knowing it will help other young doctors make their way into the world of medicine.

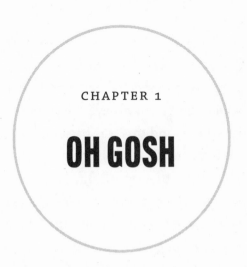

CHAPTER 1

OH GOSH

IT'S THAT AWKWARD QUESTION, JUST BEFORE YOU'RE GOING to interview someone for the first time.

"Um, how do I pronounce your name?"

"Bo-gosh, rhymes with oh gosh," he said with the matter-of-fact shrug of someone who's been saying this his whole life.

I was sitting in the Vancouver studio of *The National*, speaking for the first time to an infectious disease doctor in Toronto whose name I'd never heard, about a virus I knew almost nothing about. It was Friday, January 24, 2020. Less than a month since an alert was sent to doctors about a pneumonia of "unknown origin" in a place most of us couldn't find on a map: Wuhan, China.

Dr. Isaac Bogoch was in our studio in Toronto, looking into the camera, hearing my questions through an earpiece. It's not the most natural environment for an interview, especially for a complex story that a lot of people are worried about.

Most guests are nervous when they sit in that chair, and that includes a lot of experienced journalists. But Bogoch was relaxed, affable and seemed happy to be doing the interview. Believe me, that's not always the case when we get an expert in the studio (and this was back in the pre-pandemic days when guests actually came into studios).

Once we began the recording, I was struck by how smoothly everything went. My first ever Covid question, by the way, was "How contagious is this virus?" I was apparently very astute because Bogoch responded: "That's a great question . . ." He continued, "We still don't have the answer to that. We know it's contagious enough to be transmitted from person to person, but the question of how easily it can be transmitted from person to person still remains unknown."

From there, I asked what impact the virus has on infected people, how deadly it is, what symptoms we should be watching for in Canada, and even policy questions like why the World Health Organization hadn't yet declared this a global health emergency. The answers were quick, clear and concise. If we had any doubt about how much appetite there was for this information, it went away when we posted the interview online and got hundreds of thousands of views in the first couple of days.

A year later I watched that interview again, and there were a couple of things that made me laugh. First, when I thanked him for doing the interview, he replied, "Oh, any time." I know that's just an expression (kind of like "that's a great question"). But on that Friday night in early 2020, I wonder if Dr. "Bo-gosh" had any idea how many times we'd come calling. The second thing was at the end of our tape, in a portion that would not have aired, I started saying something like "That was exceptional." I've interviewed a lot of people—thousands for sure—in lots of settings and on lots of topics. From that first interaction, Bogoch stood out. Soon he would be joined by other doctors across the country, willing to share their expertise, generous with their time, comfortable in front of the camera, bringing just the right balance of evidence-based answers and practical advice.

From early reports in Wuhan, to the *Diamond Princess* cruise ship in Japan, to the agonizing stories from Italian hospitals, to the virus hitting North America, I've never seen a story where people had so much interest over such a long time. But that sustained interest wasn't surprising.

In one way or another, we would all feel the pandemic's impact. The tragic deaths in long-term care. The social isolation and anxiety for many people. Job losses, travel restrictions and intense need for information. The questions seemed limitless: Is it safe to walk outside? What should I do with my groceries when I get back home? What sort of mask should I wear?

In January 2020 the questions were still pretty rudimentary. Just two days after that first interview, we took Bogoch up on his offer and called him back to our studio. The first "presumptive" case in Ontario had been announced the day before. In our coverage of stories, words matter, and we were careful to add that adjective—presumptive— to every reference to that case. But in an example of the common-sense guidance we would get throughout the pandemic, Bogoch, in the interview, put "presumptive" in perspective: "That basically means the initial test done at the provincial laboratory was positive, and then they were going to send the sample to the national laboratory in Winnipeg for confirmatory testing. We knew, though, yesterday, from the first positive tests from the provincial lab—and the microbiologists will kill me for saying this—really and truly that was going to be a positive case when it went to Winnipeg, but we still had to call it presumptive until it was actually confirmed."

On the day between those *National* segments, Susy Hota, a colleague of Bogoch's at Toronto's University Health Network, did an interview with Natasha Fatah, my colleague on CBC News Network. Among the questions: What impact did this virus have on people who got infected? How can we stop the spread? When Hota was asked about rumours coming out of China that said the number of people in hospital and the number of deaths were much higher than the numbers being reported, she gave advice that would be relevant at any point during the pandemic: "It is important for people to look at credible sources of information—so official sites and official numbers—because there's a lot going around on social media and other channels that are not necessarily trustworthy and can cause alarm."

And when Fatah followed up with a question about panic, Hota's answer revealed one of the key motivations for all the doctors who were stepping forward: "I think being informed, and being informed by people who know what's going on, is incredibly important, and I think it's coming down to people like myself, who are in the middle of this, to give people the honest opinion about what's going on and to let people know we are preparing. Fear is never helpful. Panic is never helpful in a situation like this, but having a cautious approach and being prepared is what we're trying to do."

Hota remembers that day and the feeling she had as she entered the studio. "So many times in this pandemic," she says, "when you're walking into an interview and you only have a little bit of information and you're going to be in the hot seat, you've got to really be prepared to deliver the message about what you do know well."

Sometimes it was the breaking-news "hot seat," but sometimes (and pardon this metaphoric stretch) it was the more relaxing CBC Radio chesterfield. Hota was one of the many doctors who took up our invitation to spend ninety minutes on Sunday afternoons to "appear" on *Cross Country Checkup*. Two Toronto-area doctors, Zain Chagla and Sumon Chakrabarti, also answered our Sunday afternoon calls, in addition to all their appearances on CBC Television and other media outlets. So did Lynora Saxinger, from Edmonton, who on various national programs provided an important outside-of-Greater Toronto perspective on the pandemic.

As a journalist based in British Columbia, I was acutely aware the pandemic was playing out differently in various regions of the country. Same virus, different public health response. That's why I appreciated getting the perspectives of doctors outside southern Ontario: from Saxinger, of course, and, periodically, from Srinivas Murthy in Vancouver and Lisa Barrett in Halifax, a pair of Newfoundlanders who had worked across the country and around the world before landing on opposite coasts.

Murthy, in fact, is the only member of this group I've actually met. As in, I've seen him in person, not just an image on a monitor or voice in my earpiece. Before the pandemic was declared, when our newsroom was full of people, Murthy came in a few times for interviews. And on Thursday, March 12, when this sort of thing was still allowed, I went to a boardroom in BC Children's Hospital to interview him.

Pulling that tape more than a year later was fascinating. The interview was part of a longer piece about how Washington State was in crisis mode while in British Columbia, life was still going on as normal. Murthy, in the story, shared our surprise at the contrast that week between Vancouver and Seattle, less than a three-hour drive apart. "It is striking. You see cities that are so close to each other, and their demographics are so similar to each other, and yet we see very different outbreaks." There were two clips from Murthy in my story, the traditional short excerpts from a longer, pre-recorded interview. But our coverage pattern was changing, and soon Q & A sessions with doctors became an on-air staple.

In all, these doctors appeared on CBC's *The National* hundreds of times. And that's just one show, on one network. I've lost track of how often I've walked past the bank of monitors in the Vancouver newsroom, or glanced up at the TV in a coffee shop, and seen one of them on the screen, sometimes—gasp!—on a competing network!

I was astonished by how willing they were to add these interviews to their already busy lives. Fortunately, with almost everything switching to remote work from home, the doctors no longer had to take the time to come to the studio. But I'll let you in on a secret. Even when the interview is on Zoom or FaceTime, and a TV producer tells you, "We only need you for five minutes," that's not even close to being true. I don't mean the producer is trying to mislead you. It's just that by the time the control room connects with you, and we gently suggest your family might not appreciate the low angle of the laptop camera, and the director patiently asks the anchor to maybe put a little more powder on his shiny face (just a hypothetical), it's already more like ten minutes.

And this is probably after the initial brief contact with the producer, then a longer follow-up (the pre-interview), where we describe what we're looking for and learn what the doctor is in a position to talk about, while keeping open the possibility the interviewer might go in a completely different direction (or so I've heard).

To add to the degree of difficulty, the topic is a global pandemic, and you're being asked to give a few hundred thousand people advice they will then pass on to their friends and that may live forever online. Oh, and one last thing. Don't look at the image of the news anchor on your screen. Focus on that small camera lens at the top of your laptop and emote as if you're chatting with someone across a desk. Except, that's Canada peering into your home.

And be warned. Not only will what you say be closely ana-lyzed by people craving information, and perhaps by others spoiling for a fight (aerosolization, anyone?). Some will obsess about your word choice ("did she say 'disenheartening'?") or your hair. Or their perception of how tired you seem.

Thousands of people will be taking note of what's behind you. In the case of the infectious disease doctors, this was everything from Barrett's huge painting (which gets its own fan mail in the Maritimes) to Chakrabarti's carefully curated guitar cases (I think his musical hero will surprise you), Bogoch's globe (when I suggested it would make a great charity auction item, he exclaimed, "What a great idea"—then realized it belonged to his wife) and Saxinger's plant, which she placed behind her after I joked, off-air, about the starkness of the blank wall.

As you consider the content and your performance, you also have to take into account the unyielding, artificial time constraint of television.

Producer: "Could we do three questions?"

Doctor (Without hesitation): "No problem."

Producer: "In ninety seconds?"

Doctor (Thinking, pause): "Sure."

Have you ever tried to answer three questions in ninety seconds? On a sensitive, important topic? Usually for *The National* we were able to record the "hits" before the live broadcast. Often the first take would go a little long, maybe a minute fifty. In the real world that's twenty extra seconds. In the world of a newscast lineup editor it's an eternity. So we'd ask the doctor to do it again.

When I mentioned to Bogoch that the assistant director (AD) could give him counts in his earpiece, he said,

"Sure." One night, one of my favourite but slightly loud ADs hit the word "Thirty" with a little too much enthusiasm. I could see a slight flutter in Bogoch's eye as he heard her voice but wasn't exactly sure what she had said. He stumbled, or at least as close to a stumble as he would ever make during our chats. Afterward, I apologized about the distraction, and then *he* apologized for not taking the count more smoothly and said he'd be happy to do it again. Accepting counts in your ear and then offering to do it again because someone watching frame-by-frame might be able to detect a slight distraction at the one-minute mark? This is next-level guest behaviour.

But, honestly, I can't think of a single time when any of the doctors seemed reluctant to try a second take. I say "seemed" because maybe they were reluctant, but they didn't show it. Even when it was the anchor who botched the question. Even when our director—quite rightly a stickler for good audio—gently but firmly insisted a doctor find and set up a better microphone. Even when one of the doctors took a rare weekend in cottage country (when travel was allowed) and drove around to find the outer limits of cell service, then stood in a field for the interview (and, if I remember correctly, was bitten by some sort of insect mid-interview).

And through it all, they didn't shy away from questions, big, small or repeated month after month. The answers were always based on the best available information at the time. As far back as mid-March 2020, what seems like ages ago, Bogoch was asked about a particular vaccine. His answer: "It's good news about the progress, the trial shows it was safe and, in some cases, created antibodies, but this is still very early. It's a phase one trial."

Around the same time, Chagla was asked if it was safe to get groceries. At that point, not much was known about transmission. Some experts might have chosen the ultra-cautious route and said that we know very little so be very concerned. But people need to get food, and Chagla gave clear, matter-of-fact advice about choosing "a less busy grocery store, off hours," and maintaining "two-metre spacing."

I remember Saxinger being asked in May 2020 whether it was safe to have someone come into your house to clean if they took public transit to get there. That called for a fairly complex risk analysis, with the studio clock ticking. She quickly cited a study of transmission in various settings, including transit, making reference to the numbers, and then concluded, for the national audience, "It depends on your community . . . and level of community risk . . . The risk is not zero, but it's not extremely high." She wasn't avoiding the question but very efficiently pointed out there was not a definitive answer—though it can be relatively safe—while guiding viewers to determine their own answer depending on where they lived and what their personal risk tolerance was.

Then there are the contentious issues. That fall, Saxinger and Chakrabarti were on a panel dealing with the extent to which Covid is transmitted among students in schools. The question to Chakrabarti was pointed: "Is the Covid threat in schools overblown?" He later told me that he had learned school transmission was a "hot-button" topic which triggered angry criticism almost every time he addressed it.

But in this interview he didn't flinch, answering the question by going through a quick analysis: "Of course there are going to be cases [of transmission]," but there had been few, and in each documented case, transmission was not widespread. His conclusion, supported by the data at the time but highly controversial among some people, was that schools were not driving the spread of Covid in a community but, rather, reflected the spread happening more widely.

In early 2021, two more infectious disease doctors were starting to make regular appearances, at least on the shows I was hosting: Alex Wong, in Regina, and Fatima Kakkar, in Montreal. I was pleased when they accepted my invitation to be part of this book. Besides bringing perspectives from two more provinces, their stories added to what has become a very diverse narrative.

By the way, the first time I interviewed Wong and Kakkar on *The National*, I tweeted out how two more doctors were keeping up the tradition of infectious disease (ID) docs being great communicators. Every reply—and you can't often say this about Twitter—was positive.

A doctor wrote:

> I think ID docs are good at communicating because of our patients—many vulnerable folks with diverse backgrounds, languages and education. Makes it a job requirement to simplify concepts and get to what's important, while respecting people's intelligence.

Among the other comments:

> One theory: lots of practice? I can imagine
> how much of their lives is spent explaining
> diseases of all types to non-scientists.
> Popular at cocktail parties.

> They learn early on to take a great patient
> history. I guess it includes listening and
> clearly stating what they need to know.

> As a spouse to an ID doc they have to explain
> things you can't see and their tools are
> generally drugs so they have to explain side
> effects and drug interactions.

As the pandemic continued and I spent more time on the air with these doctors, I became increasingly curious about them. Given how busy they clearly were, and how much demand there was from other media and community organizations, why did they keep accepting our invitations? They never got a T-shirt or a mug. I'm sure being on TV didn't increase their business: their waiting lists were already long, even before the pandemic started.

Sometimes, on other stories, guests will make requests—they'll ask us to mention their books or display their Twitter handles. I don't mind that. As long as their answers are honest and informative, I see nothing wrong with a little brand-building. (Feel free to follow ME on Twitter, by the way.) But the infectious disease doctors never asked for anything other than getting their job descriptions right.

Even as their profile grew, their approach never changed. At least, not in any way I could tell. They never tried to leverage their growing value as guests and continued to appear on the programs to answer our questions, not promote an issue or set the agenda.

Over time, from a journalistic perspective, I realized we were witnessing an unusual phenomenon. This group of doctors was putting science front and centre during a time when evidence-based analysis was critical and when so much misinformation and disinformation on Covid was being propelled by social media, often spreading faster than the most transmissible variants. Sometimes the misinformation was promoted by scientists who were advocating a single point of view with a degree of recklessness that seemed obvious to some of us but was embraced by people who agreed with them.

These infectious disease doctors were different. This may surprise some people, but I think one of the best indicators of their approach was when, over time, some of their points turned out to be wrong. That's because the scientific understanding of Covid did change over time, at least in some areas, such as risk from surfaces (as many of us learned a new word, "fomite").

And maybe in all of this, beyond learning more about the pandemic, our collective respect for and understanding of science was being elevated. Never before have so many doctors been in the spotlight, guiding the national conversation.

I hope their diligence and reliance on data rubbed off. I also think this particular group showed us how medicine is both science AND art, using data as the foundation but also interpreting it in the real world, based on what they were seeing in patients and in the wider community.

I wonder if, in a few years, we'll see the social impact of all these media appearances. I recently heard a doctor on a podcast talking about how he and some of his peers were inspired as teenagers by the program ER, even though it stuffed six months of Hollywood emergency room drama into one prime-time hour. Is it possible that watching a group of smart, articulate men and women of different ethnicities, from across the country, explain Covid week after week for more than a year will inspire a generation of students to study science and medicine and infectious diseases? (Or name their children Sumon and Lynora?)

I also hope their work has an impact on experts in other fields. I have spent so many hours, on so many stories, trying to coax people to offer their analysis on television or radio. It is so critical to have people with real-world experience and insight give us their perspective on important stories, like criminal and aviation investigations. But experts in this country are frequently reluctant to step forward. Sometimes those who do will tell me how their colleagues treat those who speak to the media with disdain.

Often, in these other stories, we are forced to turn to US analysts, who are quick to jump in and easy to work with. I appreciate their help but I'm frustrated we can't hear Canadian voices. Not only are some issues different here—policing, for example—but seeing experts from across this country points out to people that expertise exists here. With Covid, it has been so important to have analysis based on what is happening in Edmonton or Hamilton or Halifax, rather than New York and Los Angeles.

As I worked on this book, it was a pleasure to finally learn a little more about these nine doctors, although, ever aware of their busy schedules, the phone calls were never long enough. I've joked we should have an infectious disease doctor appreciation party after all this is over. Maybe on a tropical island somewhere. (At least I would know what vaccines I'd need.)

But before that (and to be clear, there will be no party on a tropical island), this is a chance to get to know them a little better: their backgrounds, their career paths and what it's been like to suddenly be thrust from anonymity into the spotlight, becoming household names when so many Canadians were confined to their homes, desperate for information.

I don't know if there's a firm that tracks this, but the total number of media appearances by these doctors, and their cumulative audience, must be staggering. I wondered, do they get stopped on the street? Asked for advice when they buy groceries? If this was the United States, I'm sure agents would be calling with TV show or podcast ideas. What about here in Canada?

As you'll see, the nine doctors make up a fascinatingly wide-ranging group of Canadians, born from coast to coast, from Vancouver to Old Perlican, Newfoundland. Most of the interviews took place during the third wave of the pandemic, in spring of 2021, squeezed between appointments or meetings, complicated by time zones.

They answered questions without hesitation and with a high level of trust. No one asked to see anything before it went to print. As you read, imagine someone chatting on the phone rather than writing a ponderous, guarded, carefully vetted statement. This is a series of conversations, not a stack of depositions.

When you see references to family or ethnicity, it's because they brought it up. I began with the same open-ended question—tell me about yourself and your background—and let the doctors take the interview wherever they wanted. At first I had worried that profiles of nine Canadians of roughly the same age, with essentially the same jobs, would contain too many similarities. But it quickly became clear everyone's story was different. Of course, they all had one thing in common: exceptional academic achievement, though none of them talked about it until I asked them directly, and even then they often described it in a self-effacing way. Still, like the stories of hockey players spending hours at the neighbourhood rink, I thought it might be instructive to learn about the paths of some of Canada's best and brightest. Sometimes, as you'll see, success came with a few surprising detours.

I know nine people is hardly a scientific sample. But I still saw some patterns that were notable: the expectations of their families; the sometimes meandering path to medicine. Many of these motivated, accomplished students chose to do their undergrad studies in their hometowns. This still launched them on careers that took them to faraway corners of the world. And while we know them because of Covid, they've been deeply involved and motivated by many of the other great medical challenges of our time: hepatitis C, HIV/AIDS, Ebola, Zika. Work they've done on those illnesses helped prepare them for what we confronted in 2020.

I am always careful to refer to them as "Doctor" on the air, to make their expertise clear. It took a while for me to take them up on their invitation to call them by their first names in private conversations. For the purpose of this book, I'll use a combination of first, last and full names.

I know there are many more doctors who answered the media's calls. But Drs Barrett, Bogoch, Chagla, Chakrabarti, Hota, Kakkar, Murthy, Saxinger and Wong are the ones I spoke to most often. Let's begin, in alphabetical order, with a little background.

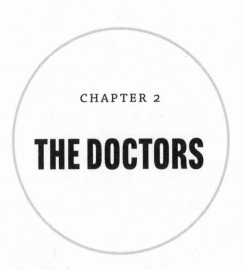

CHAPTER 2

THE DOCTORS

DR. LISA BARRETT MD, PhD, FRCPC

Clinician Scientist, Infectious Diseases
Assistant Professor, Microbiology and Immunology, Dalhousie
University

LISA BARRETT'S FIRST WORKING EXPERIENCE AT A HOSPITAL involved filing X-rays and helping out in a lab. That might not seem too surprising, except for this: she was just ten years old!

Barrett grew up in Old Perlican, Newfoundland. Population: 700.

As she explains, with a deep, throaty laugh that punctuates much of our conversation, "It was the fortunate fishing village that had the hospital AND the grocery store AND the fish plant." Both of her parents worked at the hospital. "It was a cottage hospital, the kind of place where if there was no one to babysit, you tucked your kids into the kitchen with the cook."

Her mother, Juanita, became the hospital adminis-trator; her dad, George, was an X-ray and lab tech. Barrett helped her dad file X-rays on Sunday night. She loved "the lab part of things" and remembers the thrill of running the "complete blood count machine. You put a little drop of blood in there, you push a button and it automatically does all the fancy stuff inside. I got to push the button. It was great." And it helped make it clear to pre-teen Lisa that science and medicine were her calling.

She and her sister, Mandy, went to St John's to finish high school. Lisa laughs. "My mom ripped me from my social network, not that it was much of a network. I wouldn't say I was an outgoing kid. My sister was socially awesome. I was . . ." she pauses, "the slightly less awesome one."

Though she says high school in the big city "wasn't super fun," it did provide at least one exceptional opportunity: a co-op program in medicine. Two or three afternoons a week, she and another student got to work in a lab and hang out with a professor of immunology at Memorial University's faculty of medicine. "He taught me the basics of science and inquiry and gave us this project, making holes in blood cells to make them capable of making monoclonal antibodies."

I ask her to explain the process to a non-scientist like me.

"Monoclonal antibodies have become a huge therapeutic domain—for example, we use one now for Covid treat-ment. The way you make them is you basically immortalize a cell, and to do that you poke little holes in a living cell. Not so many holes that you kill it, but enough that you

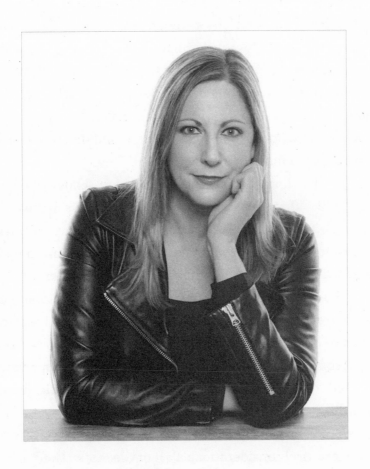

Dr. Lisa Barrett, Halifax.
Photo courtesy of Dr. Lisa Barrett

can get things into it. We were trying to look at a different way of getting those holes into living cells. The supervisor had us putting electricity through chicken red blood cells. Because we were high school students, we couldn't work with human samples because of the HIV risk and all at the time. That was a very big deal back then. We were learning how to ask questions and trying to make the right-sized holes in living cells to be able to go on and do monoclonal antibody production."

By the time she graduated from high school, she had no doubt: "That's it, I'm going to be a clinician scientist, do research and look after patients." She didn't have to travel far, beginning what would become a long association with the local university, Memorial (MUN). She says her mother was shocked she stuck around so close to home. "She tells this story a lot, about how when I was five or six, I wanted to go to boarding school. I wanted to be sent away. Did not want to live in Old Perlican. I had read up in encyclopedias, I wanted to go to boarding school. I had this romantic idea of boarding school."

As a teenager considering university, though, there were more practical considerations. Part of the motivation to stay in Newfoundland was cost. "I couldn't bear the thought, even with scholarships, of costing my parents a lot of money. They weren't poor, but they certainly weren't rich. And I'm, like, whatever. The first four years can be anywhere."

Turns out she thrived at Memorial, building strong relationships with research mentors and the administration in both biology and medicine through different activities.

And that made a persuasive case for staying at MUN. "In a way, I hated the idea of leaving that investment."

At the same time, just off the campus, she was getting a different but equally formative education, which she describes as "probably the best thing I ever did." That seminal experience for the young woman on a path to her PhD and medical degree? Working at the Guv'nor Pub for four or five years. She says it was just like the bar in the TV show *Cheers*. Everyone knew everyone else, and it helped transform the self-described "awkward nineteen-year-old." Barrett says people sometimes tell her, "'You talk so well. Must have been all those speeches in school.' And yes, I did a lot of public speaking in high school, but I really credit Guv'nor."

After undergrad she spent another year on campus, doing research, and then applied to a single medical school: Memorial. She got in, but it didn't feel quite right.

"I began to wonder, did I really want to go to medical school? I still loved research so much, so I thought, 'What about a combined PhD/MD program?' Problem was, Memorial didn't offer a combined program. So I thought, 'Why not make one?'"

The dean of the medical school was Ian Bowmer, an infectious disease (ID) doctor and HIV researcher. Barrett, Bowmer and her PhD supervisor, Michael Grant, wrote the rules and regulations for a new program, which they submitted to the university senate. The senate said yes.

After getting that combined degree, it was time to continue her education beyond Newfoundland. Barrett looked at "six or seven" internal medicine residencies across the country. She says she was very interested in the University of British Columbia, and included Dalhousie University, in Halifax, almost as an afterthought. But it was there that an ID doctor, Lynn Johnston, made what turned out to be a persuasive pitch. (Infectious diseases is one of the sub-specialties of internal medicine, which also includes specialties like cardiology, immunology and geriatric medicine.)

"She knew me from HIV research conferences, and she said, 'Lisa, you and I should chat.' And she is a Wonder Woman. Huge contributor to ID in Canada. She sat me down and said, 'You should come to Dal to do your internal medicine.' I thought, 'Oh, okay.' And then she said, 'You're going to come back here after you do your ID, when you go away and do other stuff, and then we're going to get you a job as a clinician scientist. There aren't many of those, but I want someone on my team in a few years who's strong on research. We're making a long-term plan here.' So after a big cross-country tour, I decided to go to Dal and they accepted me."

After residency, it was off to Toronto for an infectious diseases fellowship—training with one of the other doctors in this book, Sumon Chakrabarti. Along the way, there were what Barrett casually refers to as "some delays in my training." One happened in Vancouver, when she was taking a medical school elective course.

"I couldn't breathe. I was running in Point Grey [a neighbourhood near the University of British Columbia campus] and realized, 'I think I have a heart problem.' I asked a doctor to take a listen. I had blown one of my heart valves." Barrett mentions this as matter-of-factly as if she were describing a broken pipe in her house. "I took six weeks off to have a heart valve fixed," and then it was back to work.

In a follow-up call, I ask if she could tell me more about what happened. "Yeah, it was significant," she says. "I was basically in mild heart failure for a couple of months until I went back to get it looked after. The thing about being young is that your body is amazing and can tolerate lots of disturbance before it calls it quits, but, yeah, that was significant."

She left Vancouver and returned home to Newfoundland, where a doctor set her up with a heart surgeon in Toronto. "He was one of the people who developed this surgical technique to fix the mitral valve. He was the world leader in this repair so they didn't have to replace the valve. The thought is at some point, likely as I get older, it will need to get repaired again or replaced, but at the moment—because my friend is a cardiologist and she made me get a heart echo a couple of weeks ago—it looks beautiful."

As I interviewed the ID doctors for this book, I discovered lots of surprises in their stories, and connections to other ID doctors. In Barrett's case, that includes working at the National Institutes of Health (NIH) in Bethesda, Maryland, with Dr. Anthony Fauci. He was then, as he is now, the director of a branch of the NIH called the National Institute of Allergy and Infectious Disease (NIAID).

Barrett says there is a MUN connection to how she ended up at NIAID: Shyam Kottilil, a medical doctor who got his PhD in immunology in St John's. Barrett knew him from when she was an undergrad. She reached out to Kottilil about the possibility of working in Bethesda, and in a sentence that almost certainly sums up a more complicated process, Barrett tells me, "He said sure, come on down!"

She jokes, "All Fauci knew was that I was from Canada, and he knew about Labrador because he went salmon fishing up there a few times." Beyond that, I was curious what insights she had from working with the doctor who took on such a critical leadership role in the US during the pandemic.

Did she hang out with Fauci? "No one really hangs out with him. If you did, it's because you were doing something wrong. He likes to give people their room, just provide a little guidance. Don't get in the weeds, keep it high level. And he'll ask you a few key questions, 'What are you really going to make of this data?' But mainly his approach was hands off, big picture."

She offers this example: In her last year at the NIH, before she returned to Halifax, she went to a 7,000-person conference in Europe. "It was a time when the first really and truly curative drugs for hepatitis C were coming to the market. The rate of clearance and cure was very high. We were doing clinical trials on people who were co-infected with HIV and hepatitis C, and this was some of the first data that showed these patients could be treated and cured just as easily, and my specific project was looking at the immune response. It was the first data being presented, pretty much in the world, on these drugs and demonstrating your immune system recovers after this."

In what seems like pretty good training for a woman who would one day help Nova Scotians deal with a pandemic, Barrett says Fauci had high expectations but also a high degree of faith. He told her, "I'm not going to look at your slides until the day before, and I won't provide much advice."

"That's what he expected," she tells me, "that we would do it the way it needed to be done, and if we couldn't, someone else could do it for us."

DR. ISAAC I. BOGOCH, MS, FRCPC, DTM&H

Staff Physician, Infectious Diseases, Toronto General Hospital
Associate Professor, Department of Medicine, University
    of Toronto

IT'S NOT LONG INTO OUR FIRST PHONE CALL BEFORE IT becomes clear that Isaac Bogoch is upbeat. Irrepressibly. Almost, but not quite, unbelievably. In the space of forty minutes he uses the word "great" or "wonderful" more than twenty times. The city of Calgary? "I really, really love the city. A wonderful place to grow up." Undergrad at the University of Calgary? "Best time of my life." Technically, that can't be true because here's how he describes a long trip he took before medical school to Southeast Asia and Australia: "Best year of my life." Like I said, upbeat.

And here's the thing: that's the Bogoch I've seen when we connected remotely for those countless TV interviews during the pandemic. Or more to the point, the way he was even when he was off camera. That's not insignificant. Over the years I've done lots of interviews with people who went

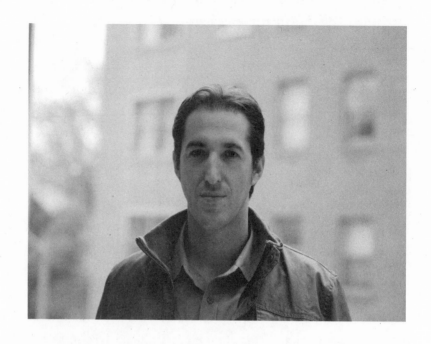

Dr. Isaac Bogoch, Toronto.
Photo courtesy of Dr. Isaac Bogoch

from grumpy to affable to grumpy as the red "On Air" light went on and off. Not Isaac.

I'll let his family decide if his sunny disposition led to success or vice versa, but his life does seem to have been pretty good. He says he had a "modest upbringing. My mom [Renee] was a teacher, my dad [Milton] a small business owner. I've got an older brother and a younger sister." He loved Calgary because it had "lots of nature, lots of places to ride your bike. I just basically remember being outside for the first twenty years of my life. I really do love the city."

His two main interests growing up? Hockey and science. He says if he was watching TV as a kid, he'd likely put down the remote when he got to *Hockey Night in Canada* or "David Attenborough narrating as some crocodile ate a poor impala who had just been getting a sip of water. I'd always end up on those two channels.

"I really liked the sciences. I knew I was going to do something science related, even in high school. I was always attracted to that. I always liked natural history. I could try to make it academic and explain it's because of this, this and this, but in reality, I don't really know. It's just what I'd gravitate towards, it's interesting, and I somehow ended up integrating that into a career so I was pretty happy about that."

He played hockey at a fairly competitive level—Double A teams—until he graduated from high school, when he decided it was time to scale down that part of his life. "I was decent but clearly not good enough to get a good scholarship, but some of my teammates went pretty far. I had some terrible offers to try out for terrible schools with terrible scholarships and I didn't even bother." But he did keep playing, in recreational leagues. "I've played hockey in every year of my life since I was five." He pauses for a moment. "Well, except the pandemic."

The end of his competitive hockey career didn't mean Bogoch was ready to devote his life to that other passion, science. Finishing high school a semester early, he took on a couple of jobs to save some money: skate sharpening at a pro shop and assisting a butcher by carrying slabs of meat. Then, at the age of seventeen, he bought a ticket to Europe to travel before starting undergrad studies at the University of Calgary. "My family didn't have much money, so I lived at home." And when he started, he admits that "in the balance of school, friends and fun, I definitely tilted towards friends and fun."

In a story that will likely sound familiar to lots of people, the first term of first year was a bit of an adjustment. "I probably spent a little too much time at the campus pub," he admits, and, being an eighteen-year-old in Calgary, when the local ski conditions were good, he and his friends would head off to the mountains.

It would be a nice dramatic turn to say he failed the year and needed to start over. Not quite.

In the first semester his grades "were good but not medical school good," but that quickly changed. "I realized if I was going to pursue a career in academics, either with medicine or science, I had to pick it up."

Even when he concentrated on improving his grades, though, "I still had a wonderful time. I look fondly on my time at the University of Calgary. I loved it. I mean, you look at the *Maclean's* ranking [of Canadian universities], it's always twenty-third out of twenty-four schools or something. I don't care. I had wonderful, wonderful teachers, wonderful people that I'm still very close with—these were my science mentors at the time—and some of the best friends I made along the way.

"I spent time doing research not just in labs but also ecological settings. In my undergrad I did a really cool course in Belize where we were studying howler monkeys. I thought eventually, if I pursued science, it would be a combination of lab work and field work." But by the time he graduated, he decided he would go into medicine. After another detour.

"I'd been in school a long time, right? I wasn't ready to go into anything. I knew medical school was going to be a big deal, it was going to be a lot of work, and I didn't even apply. I took a pause and saved up some money working in a lab." He took a year off, finally filled out some applications, and then bought a plane ticket to Kenya, spending six months "travelling around East Africa and Southern African with a tent and just hanging out and seeing things I always wanted to see."

Periodically he'd check back with his parents to find out if any of the medical schools he'd applied to had written back. When he found out four had offered him interviews, he cut his trip short and returned to Canada. But after doing the interviews, instead of waiting to hear whether he would be accepted, he was off again. He worked for a couple of months and convinced a friend, one of his old hockey teammates, to travel with him to Southeast Asia. He was in Australia when his parents gave him the news over the phone: a letter of acceptance had arrived from the University of Toronto.

You might think his response would be simple: say yes and head to Toronto. Apparently not.

"The first reaction was 'that's great, that's amazing. I can be a doctor.' But the next thing that came to mind was 'I'm in Brisbane having the time of my life. I got in once. I probably can get in again.' I was thinking maybe I should take another year off and continue surfing, but I was broke, didn't have a cent to my name, and I thought maybe it is time."

The logistics of moving to Toronto were easy. There wasn't much to pack. But for a kid from the west, the shift in culture was more significant. Bogoch says Toronto was "a completely different world, not just a different city but a very different mentality, and that was a huge, huge change."

Add to that the challenge of medical school. Bogoch says—no surprise—he quickly embraced it. "I worked like a dog. Made some wonderful friends and I really came to love the city of Toronto. You sort of think, 'Are you in the right place at the right time with the right people?' And I truly was."

He says that applied to his four years of internal medicine residency in Toronto as well. "I just had a big group of wonderful, supportive and fun friends. The hours are crazy. You really work hard. You think medical school is tough, residency is tougher."

Bogoch says time off was rare and precious. "I had a great group of people who were fun and open-minded and adventurous, and if we stuck around in Toronto, we'd do fun things in the city like go to restaurants you wouldn't normally think about or find great mountain biking trails that, if you weren't from here, you wouldn't know existed."

As for specializing in infectious diseases, that decision came later. Bogoch admits it was almost a process of elimination. "I liked a lot of things in medical school." An elective in trauma surgery during the Calgary Stampede? "It was really interesting and I had a lot of fun but I recognized early on I probably wouldn't be a surgeon." Pediatrics? "Loved it." But—"Not for me." Obstetrics/gynecology? "When you're on these rotations, so much of your experience is based on who you're with. And I was with the world's best obstetricians and gynecologists. I had the best time on the rotation. I remember thinking, as a medical student, 'Maybe I'll do this. I'm having a wonderful time.' And then you wake up one day and say, 'What, are you nuts? I don't want to do this with my life.' I loved the people I was working with, but it's probably not the profession for me."

Choosing a residency in internal medicine allowed him to defer the decision on what to specialize in. "I really liked intensive care medicine. I liked respirology and I liked infectious diseases." He says he eventually settled on infectious diseases, in part, because it complemented his interest in global health, travelling to West Africa and South Asia. He also liked the lifestyle. "I knew I didn't want to live in the hospital. I can't say that with a straight face in 2020 or 2021, but I wanted to have a life. I wanted to have a family, work hard, but I have a lot of interests outside of medicine and I didn't want to ignore that."

He did his infectious diseases fellowship at Harvard, and then a master's in public health before deciding to return to Toronto. His fiancée, now wife, moved down with him and they had their first child. "It was a very special few years down there. I had a wonderful time, they're very supportive. You hear a lot of things about Harvard, it could be competitive or snooty. And honestly, none of that was true. World-class clinicians. World-class scientists. Wonderful, wonderful people."

Two more notes about Bogoch. The second time I interview him, I mention how many superlatives he used to describe his friends and his experiences over the years. He chuckles and says I can probably chalk it up to the caffeine he'd just had. "I usually have lots of energy, but when I'm tired I sometimes turn to coffee, and then I'm more annoying than usual."

And he also told me a story about a couple of less than excellent moments that played a role in his going to medical school in Toronto rather than Alberta, which he was leaning toward. He applied to both med schools in his home province, but the interviews, by his own admission, didn't go well. "I'm not blaming anyone but myself," he says, laughing. He'd just returned from his Africa adventure and was "a little rusty." Adding to that, the morning he went to Edmonton, he cut himself shaving.

During the interview, it felt like the cut was starting to bleed again. Imagine being a young, prospective medical school student. This interview could well be a pivotal moment in your life, and you're pretty sure a trickle of blood is forming on your upper lip. Bogoch says rather than acknowledging it, perhaps even joking about it, he chose a different approach, placing his hand on his face for the rest of the interview.

"As I walked out of the interview, I thought, 'That didn't go badly.' But as I was driving back to Calgary, I'm somewhere near Red Deer, playing this interview over and over in my head, and I thought, 'OH MY GOD . . . that was horrible. There is no chance I'm getting into that medical school.' And I didn't. And rightly so."

DR. ZAIN CHAGLA

Infectious Diseases Physician
Medical Director of Infection Control, St Joseph's Healthcare
Associate Professor, McMaster University

IT TOOK ME A FEW INTERVIEWS BEFORE I FOCUSED ON ZAIN Chagla's lapel pin. During our tapings for *The National* I was either looking straight into the camera or glancing at him on a small monitor. But one day, after we did the interview, I walked over to the monitor to get a closer look. It was only then I noticed it wasn't a piece of jewellery or a pin denoting some sort of professional association. Instead, I realized Chagla was almost certainly the only doctor on national television who was declaring his loyalty to the Toronto Raptors every day.

That somewhat subtle homage to his beloved team seems right on brand for a guy who takes science seriously but loves basketball. Although when I ask him to describe the teenage Zain, he concedes he didn't embody the cool swagger of the NBA. "I was pretty social but I can't say I was not a geek." He pauses and then laughs. "Yeah, I was probably a geek. Pretty academically okay."

That is almost certainly an understatement. Like so many people in this book, Chagla is part of a wave of immigrants whose families came to this country because of science and whose parents instilled the pursuit of science in their children. His dad, Abdul, was a microbiologist, who got his master's degree in Karachi, Pakistan, and his PhD in Wales before moving to North America.

Years before Zain had any idea what his career choice would be, his father was connecting with some of North America's leading infectious disease experts. Abdul Chagla did his post-doctoral work in Bethesda, Maryland, interacting with Dr. Anthony Fauci, and later was at Toronto's Sick Kids Hospital. Zain says his dad's "benchmates were Donald Low and Allison McGeer," who became well known nationally when they were answering media questions and giving analysis during the SARS crisis of 2003. (Severe acute respiratory syndrome was another disease caused, like Covid, by a coronavirus, which originated in China. There were more than four hundred reported cases in Canada, and forty-four deaths, most in the Toronto region.) A few years earlier, Abdul Chagla had a role in another Canadian public health emergency when his lab was responsible for testing in Walkerton, Ontario, after *E. coli* contaminated the town's water supply in 2000, killing at least seven people.

The career path of Chagla's mother, Yasmine, was perhaps even more impressive. She worked in the home until

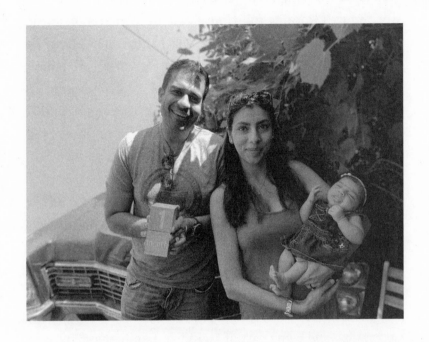

Dr. Zain Chagla with his wife, Noor Manji, and
their daughter, Kalenya Chagla, in Mississauga.
Photo courtesy of Dr. Zain Chagla

Zain and his brother were teenagers, then began pursuing her undergraduate degree in nursing. By the time he had graduated from high school, she had graduated from university and was working full-time as a nurse. You can hear the admiration in Zain's voice as he tells his mother's story: "It was very inspirational for the pursuit of learning throughout life. Not just turning it off when you get your last degree."

Born in Toronto, Chagla grew up in London, Ontario, and says his childhood was "pretty typical, playing basketball, there wasn't anything crazy. It was kind of a small town, you knew your neighbours."

He shrugs off his academic side—"I did okay"—until I press him on it. When I say he must have done well, he says, matter-of-factly, "I worked hard. My parents instilled that in me. Some people struggle with the medical sciences, but I guess I seemed to thrive in them, the ability to pick things up easily, which I'm thankful for. I'm blessed in the sense, from my upbringing and being part of an Indian family, it's something that's ingrained in you to aim for the best and keep pushing."

But, he's quick to point out, he doesn't excel in everything. "I absolutely hate writing. The medical sciences are amazing because the descriptiveness of your writing is terrible, right? You write these extremely scientific pieces that have a very regimented jargon associated with that. You don't have any expression. Your grammar can be relatively scientific. That doesn't necessarily reflect real prose. So, yeah, I was terrible at English. That creativity, creative writing, has always been something I struggle with. It's ironic that during the pandemic I started writing again quite a bit."

Chagla did his undergrad at Western University in his hometown, and by the end of his first year felt pretty sure he would eventually be a doctor. He started to volunteer at a hospital and got to know people involved in research, and he found that "fascinating"—so fascinating he applied to medical school after just three years of undergrad. He landed on the wait-list for Queen's University in Kingston, Ontario. Where he waited.

And then, a day he remembers vividly: "I was registering for fourth-year courses because I thought this [medical school] was not going to happen. I figured I needed to go and find a research project next year and work on the application a bit. I was literally booting up the computer to book fourth-year courses, and there was a note in my inbox saying, 'If you still want a spot, there's one here.'" Getting that email "was such a relief," he says now.

He enjoyed his time at Queen's. "People were really close, so it was nice in that sense. Loved the mentorship. You knew everyone. Your profs were really good role models. Some of them are people I work with today."

When I ask about what stands out, the formative experiences, Chagla tells me, "Honestly, my bigger memories are about time on the wards and the patient experiences than in the classroom. There were two things that were really eye-opening. We learn so much about the social determinants of health, how it is multifactorial, but when you start seeing it in reality of how income and employment and education affect health care, it was a slap in the face. It was very apparent that this is reality. You see it in basically every rotation, this social determinant of health piece, everything from psych to obstetrics to medicine to surgery."

It's easy to overlook how young and, to an extent, naive students can be. Chagla says that for him, as a medical student in his early twenties, the clinical part of medical school gave him his first real view of how the system works. "Health care, especially in hospitals, wasn't what TV had made it out to be. I think you have a sense that hospitals should be places where patients are cared for but, again, social situations, that transition to long-term care, bed shortages and seasonal changes, where you're just trying to get as many people out as in, it becomes so apparent how we live with a fragile health care system. Hospitals being what they are, they're places of great teamwork, great care, but they have this constant undercurrent of underfunding and health care utilization, patient movement, and it's a perspective you never really get until you're working inside the hospital."

Despite his father's connection to infectious diseases, Chagla wasn't immediately sure what specialty he'd pursue. "I was interested in pathology initially, but I missed the patient interaction. I was terrible at deep procedural stuff, and surgery was off the table quickly." As he studied internal medicine, he went through a checklist as he looked at the sub-specialties: "Could I actually live this lifestyle? Do I understand it? Would I be able to see these patients every day? And it really came back to ID. There is such a variety of things.

"There's a quote. Infectious disease doctors have to be the second-smartest doctors because you have to know every body system almost as well as the specialist in that body system, because when it gets infected, they're calling you for help. You have to know pulmonology and respirology just slightly less than a respirologist but enough to read the CAT scan and get a good sense of what's going on. You have to know obstetrics slightly less than the obstetrician to understand the complications to delivery and what that means to a fetus."

He says that's what drew him to it. "It affects every body system. You have to have a good knowledge of a number of things."

And there are the bigger issues. "It has a lot of policy stuff in terms of infection control. There's a lot of global health, which has always been a big piece of my career. And the mix between the lab and the patient. The combination of all that made it super appealing. There wasn't anything else in medicine that replicated that. Everyone's career is so different, even when they do ID."

That reference to global health is something that keeps coming up with infectious disease doctors. For Chagla, a three-month program in Tanzania and Uganda had a lasting impression. It was run by the London (UK) School of Hygiene and Tropical Medicine and drew doctors from around the world. As well, about a third of the class was from East Africa.

"When you do tropical medicine you want to see unusual parasites and cool stuff in the microscope and see interesting patients, but it was my first deep dive, a fundamental clinical experience, where you get the sense of what health care systems look like in low- and middle-income settings, some of the practical challenges of providing medical care outside of richly resourced settings. Attitudes and culture and how they interlace with medicine outside of the Western world. It was incredibly eye-opening."

Like many people who have worked in the developing world, when he returned, he struggled with what he'd seen. "What are we doing here and why are we doing it where we could be so much more efficient in our day-to-day practice in Canada."

Chagla says, "I had to sit down with a few people I had known who had similar experiences in their training or their practice and ask, 'How do you balance this? How do you go back to practising in a well-resourced Canadian context and then going back to sub-Saharan Africa or rural India and practising there or developing health systems there?'

"It's always stayed with me, as a clinician and a person, and how I approach problems. It always keeps me balanced to remember those times and remember how the rest of the world lives and practises and deals with medicine."

DR. SUMON CHAKRABARTI, MD, FRCPC, DTM&H

Infectious Diseases Physician, Trillium Health Partners,
    Mississauga site
Lecturer, University of Toronto

THINK ABOUT HOW OLD YOU WERE WHEN YOU WERE SURE what your career job would be. And then consider Sumon Chakrabarti: "I was that prototypical Indian kid whose parents wanted him to be a doctor from the very beginning.

To be a doctor, it encompasses who I am and I love doing it, and the idea was introduced to me when I was very young."

And he means it when he says very young. "I'm not kidding you. I've wanted to be a doctor since I was five years old. In my Grade 8 yearbook I put that as my dream, to become a doctor. This is actually something I have been thinking about since childhood."

Chakrabarti was born in Sarnia, where his father, Naren, was a mechanical engineer in Chemical Valley, and his mother, Dipa, was a music teacher. He says his childhood "shaped a lot of who I am today because I had a really good mix of Indian friends and non-Indian friends. From my community at the temple I had working-class friends, quote, unquote 'rich' friends. You get the picture." It was a broad, diverse group that Chakrabarti thrived in. "I was always a very outgoing person, not shy, always willing to meet people. I was very focused on academics but at the same time I was very much like my dad. Being social was a huge part of who I was."

Chakrabarti says his parents, who were from India, "were big on assimilating with Canadian culture, but at the same time very proud of our roots." He comfortably stepped between two worlds, a Sarnia kid who cheered for the Montreal Canadiens (not the obvious choice in a region where hockey loyalty was split between the Leafs and the nearby Detroit Red Wings) and who also connected to his family history, reading and speaking Bengali. "That's very much who I was . . . and who I am."

Music was also a big part of his childhood. Violin lessons first, and then, in Grade 9, inspired by a friend in school,

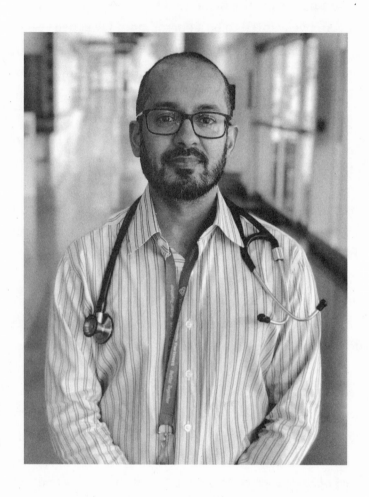

Dr. Sumon Chakrabarti, Mississauga.
Photo by Mike Hajmasy of Trillium Health Partners

guitar. "My dad bought this kind of beat-up old acoustic from a garage sale, and I never looked back. When I was in high school, I would come home and I would sit with a guitar for hours."

As with all the doctors in this book, I push him to tell me about excelling in schoolwork. "It was something that was very much ingrained in me as a kid, that you always have to be good at academics. One thing I will say, and I don't mean to brag, I just found that, for the most part, new concepts came easily to me."

He remembers in medical school there were people who would "study like crazy." He says there were some subjects he struggled with, but "I was able to balance those things without keeping my nose in the book from 9 a.m. to 9 p.m."

That childhood dream to be a doctor took on a sharper focus when he was diagnosed with nephrotic syndrome at age fourteen. He explains that it was "a kidney defect that spills a lot of protein in your urine. It can lead to kidney damage." He says, "No one knows what caused it. It may have been an allergic reaction or something else." But he took a powerful steroid, prednisone, and it worked. "It melted away and never came back. In the back of my mind I always wonder if it will come back, but I'm forty-one now and haven't had a kidney problem."

It was a good outcome that left a positive legacy. Chakrabarti says that "significant brush with the health care system" added to his interest in the medical profession, especially dealing with patients. And it left him with a more specific goal: to become a nephrologist.

From Sarnia, he did his undergrad at Western University in London, Ontario, then went on to medical school. And it was there, early in first year, that he had a bit of a culture shock. The first few months of medical school, with the intense flow of new concepts and information, "was like drinking from a firehose." Surrounded by very smart, highly motivated students, he says those early days in class were particularly suited to people who were studying all day and excelled at "rote memorization." Apparently that wasn't him. A few weeks in, Chakrabarti had his first quiz in anatomy. For a student used to getting 90s, it was "a shock. I got 63 per cent. I never got a mark that low in my life."

Eventually things turned around as he made friends and felt himself settling in. But it wasn't until third year, when he was seeing patients in hospital, that he felt more comfortable. "My knowledge base was much more applicable in a clinical setting. Being on the ward, dealing with patients, I felt that was something I was excelling at and I realized I was in the right place."

That sense of being in the right place was, he says, greatly influenced by a class with Dr. David Colby, who became one of Chakrabarti's mentors. "He started to talk about really cool things about infectious diseases. For us, as medical students, infectious diseases was really arduous. You had to remember these meticulous names of organisms and that turns you off right away." But Colby would present them with medical puzzles: "What could happen if you have a cut, you have liver disease and you go into ocean water? What bug could cause a problem?" Chakrabarti tells me the answer is *Vibrio vulnificus* aka "monster of the deep." "Or this woman, usually quiet, suddenly becomes really outgoing. She buys a whole bunch of expensive stuff, and a day later she develops meningitis." A classic case of meningococcal mania, he explains to me. "I thought, 'THIS IS REALLY COOL.'"

Solving the medical puzzles in class appealed to him and, as it turns out, had a practical application as well. "Believe it or not, a few years into my career I actually saw a case of meningococcal mania. I had thought, 'This is totally lore,' but discovering the case reinforced why I love this profession so much."

Cool perhaps, but it created a dilemma for an aspiring kidney doctor. Chakrabarti struggled with which direction to pursue. "At the last minute I chose infectious diseases. I realized it was my true love."

He says he was inspired, in part, by the late Dr. Jay Keystone, who he describes as "the guru of infectious diseases. I trained with him for a year and saw all sorts of fascinating things." Chakrabarti says that, at first, the tropical infections he had learned about seemed far away from his practice in southern Ontario, but "all of a sudden you realize in the GTA [Greater Toronto Area] we have lots of people coming from tropical areas, and you see manifestations of these illnesses here in Canada. So there's clearly a need for this. I really liked it." He has "seen multiple cases of leprosy, tons and tons of malaria, typhoid," among other things.

Chakrabarti knew he wanted to teach and see patients. He thought, "I have this niche [of skills]. Where can I use it?" The answer to that question was Mississauga, which is west of Toronto. "There's this massive hospital, massive unmet need in the community. It's been rewarding."

In the course of our interview I discover that what an infectious disease doctor considers rewarding includes "opportunities" like this: "We performed the first tapeworm cyst removal from a brain here at our hospital. The patient had the cyst in the ventricle inside her brain. Nobody had removed one of those before in Canada. I talked to one of the neurosurgeons here, he was also interested, and we did it."

That passion for tropical diseases connected him with two other doctors featured in this book. Chakrabarti was a staff doctor when he treated a patient who had been working at Toronto's food terminal. "A scorpion in a box of mangoes from Mexico bit him. He brought the scorpion to the Emergency. I helped manage that, and Zain Chagla [then a young doctor in training] was interested in writing that up. We wrote the article up together and it was published."

A few years earlier, Chakrabarti had gone to Toronto to do his internal medicine residency, feeling a little out of place in the big city. On the first day, he says, another first-year resident came up, stuck out his hand and said, "I'm Isaac Bogoch." By second year they had become friends and spent three months together studying tropical diseases in Peru. When Chakrabarti got married, Bogoch was in his wedding party, along with Chakrabarti's childhood friends from Sarnia. They included some he had known since he was that five-year-old dreaming of being a doctor.

I ask Chakrabarti if there is anything else about his pre-pandemic life I should know. He says that as disruptive as

Covid has been, he realizes he was ready for it. "The one thing about my life, it was pretty happy. I had a job, married, I have two kids. Everything at that point of time was very stable." He laughs. "Obviously this pandemic sucks. But I think that stability helped prepare me mentally for what was to come."

DR. SUSY HOTA

Infectious Diseases Specialist
Medical Director, Infection Prevention and Control, University Health Network
Associate Professor, Department of Medicine, University of Toronto

IT ISN'T EXACTLY A SECRET, BUT IT DID TAKE A COUPLE OF very specific questions to find out about Susy Hota's connection to euphoria. Or, more accurately, "You4'ya"—something that played an essential, and perhaps surprising, role in helping her become the doctor who seems so comfortable live on camera.

But let's begin where she was born, Saint-Jean-sur-Richelieu, a small city about forty kilometres southeast of Montreal. It's perhaps best known for Collège militaire royal de Saint-Jean, where her dad, Nalini Kanta Hota, who was a chemist, did research.

Hota candidly says that in the 1980s it was "not the best of times to be a visible minority there. I'll be honest and say childhood was not always the most pleasant experience."

But she and her sisters focused on their schoolwork. Her parents instilled in them that doing well in school was like a job.

By the time she was in junior high, the family had moved to the Montreal suburb of Brossard, which Hota describes as being a bit more diverse. She eventually went to a program for gifted children in Grades 7 and 8. It was "very academically focused, intense. We were in a separate stream in a large school."

And then, in Grade 9, a big shift. Her father had died when Hota was eleven, and her mother, Charulata Hota, married a geophysics professor, Lalatendu Mansinha, at Western University. They moved to London, Ontario, and Hota remembers thinking how different it was: "People are so nice here, it's so open. There were some great people in the school. In Quebec I grew up with pretty overt racism. It wasn't like that in London. I think some people had some thoughts and feelings I learned about later," she says with a laugh, "but it wasn't the same. People wouldn't come to your face and call you names."

Still, moving to a new town can be tough, and Hota worried she wasn't fitting in. "There was that feeling sometimes of 'I don't quite belong here' throughout my younger years."

Hota says she continued to focus on schoolwork, but a new academic interest had a big impact on her life. She credits a high school music teacher with helping her develop her passion for singing. Through this, she says, "I gained the confidence to step away from the shyness that was kind of the

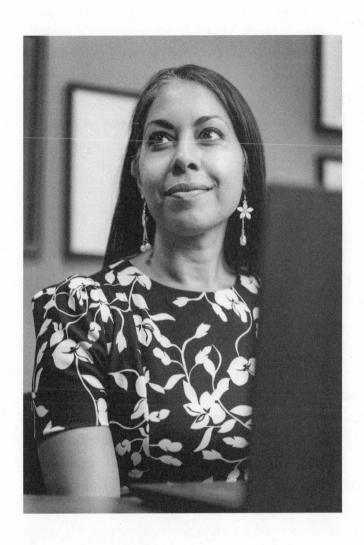

Dr. Susy Hota, Toronto.
Photo by Kyle Laurin

introverted side of me that normally would dominate, and I could actually get out there."

Hota says, "I loved listening to music, the harmonies. But on the technical side I'm not very good at reading music, writing music, none of that. I listen by ear."

And that's where You4'ya comes in, an a capella group she formed with one of her sisters and a couple of close friends. She laughs when I ask her about the group's name. "We thought it was very clever. I'm sure it was used somewhere else . . . but this was before the internet and [before] people could check on trademarks."

They would listen to songs, arrange vocals and tour some of southern Ontario's summer festivals. "We made a tiny bit of money but it was mainly for fun and to explore the artistic side of things.

"I would get nervous, yet we wanted to do it, we wanted to try and get out there. It was a way to push myself past my comfort zone. I was shy, very shy, as a kid, and you'd think this was the last thing I'd want to do. But it was exhilarating and made me recognize you can have different selves. I had my performance self, which was able to go up there and do that, and then my everyday self, which would be, like, 'Oh my God, I can't believe it.'"

Like many of the doctors in this book, Hota went to her hometown university. In her case, that was Western in London. She started in science and eventually had to make a tough decision, between chemistry—where she had her highest marks—and biology. In the end, perhaps foreshadowing a career in infectious diseases, she chose microbiology and immunology.

In a family of scientists, she considered doing a graduate degree but quickly realized that "basic science research" wouldn't be right for her. In the lab, she says, "It's frustrating to be looking so minutely at the detail and trying to figure out one piece of the puzzle. And when it doesn't go right, you just feel like maybe this is a signal I should be doing something a bit broader rather than being focused on a particular, mechanistic thing."

And so it was off to medical school at the University of Toronto. Hota says she was excited about going to the big city, but school didn't go well, at least not at first. She got that sinking feeling again, wondering if she belonged. Anatomy was not her favourite subject, she says. She didn't know any of her classmates. And some of them were competitive to a fault. When they needed hard copies of X-rays to share and study from, Hota says that some would "go missing. People would hide them. Not my style at all, not how I wanted to learn, not the environment I wanted to be in."

And then there was the first test. "I remember panicking on the first bell-ringer exam, which is a practical exam where you go from station to station and try to identify the anatomy and answer some questions. I just tried to get through that exam, and I did not do well. At all."

When she got her exam back, there were two surprises. The first was her mark: 70 per cent. "Not so bad given I was freaking out and thought I failed it," but clearly not good enough. The second surprise was a sticky note from the director of the course, informing the bottom 5 per cent that they needed to come in and see him.

She stood in line with a group of strangers, making self-deprecating jokes. She remembers chatting with one classmate and spotted his mark: 93 per cent. She thought, "Oh my God, he's probably here to try to argue he deserves a couple of extra points while the rest of us in the sticky note club are being called to the office. It was one of those 'where am I?' moments."

But things soon changed, and music played a role. In first year, Hota saw a poster for an annual Canadian Cancer Society fundraising show, Daffodil, and auditioned to become one of the singers. She ended up performing one of the solos in front of nightly audiences of a few hundred people. Hota says it was "a huge experience at the beginning of medical school that shaped how the rest of med school went."

She says she ended up "loving" the school experience and graduated in the top 10 per cent of the class, "so it goes to show the importance of sticking with it, you know. But I really felt like giving up at some points in the first three months."

As Hota did her rotations in medical school, she says she enjoyed general surgery and psychiatry, but it was internal medicine that "spoke to me from the start." It appealed to her curiosity and problem solving. "I think if I didn't do medicine, I'd do forensic science. When I was a kid I thought I would be a detective, or a private investigator. That's what I really enjoyed doing, trying to solve problems, and a lot of it is the complexity of the problems that appeal to me in internal medicine. So that was an easy-ish decision to make, and the program that was the strongest I was looking for and one of the best in the country was right here in Toronto."

She felt pulled toward gastroenterology, another sub-specialty of internal medicine, but in the end the breadth of infectious diseases won her over. "You could be someone well versed in tropical medicine, international medicine, or you could be a science researcher trying to understand the immunology of something. Again, it spoke to the bigger picture and the problem solving. And I liked the public health side of things, investigating outbreaks of infections, things like that, even at that stage."

Hota says when she left London, Ontario, for medical school, it wasn't her intention to stay in Toronto for so long. But at every point she felt the best option for her happened to be in the city, from residency to fellowship to her first job: infectious diseases physician in the infection control department at the University Health Network in Toronto.

"I stumbled into it . . . applied for it . . . got the position and thought I could do it for two years and go do something else." It turned out to be a job she loves and has continued doing. "I lucked out that way. I don't think jobs just land on people's doorsteps so easily."

Her first boss was Michael Gardam. "I thought, he's an interesting guy, and he's got a cool perspective." Hota began working four years after SARS and just as another infectious disease, *Clostridium difficile* or *C. difficile*, was hitting hospitals hard. One of her academic interests was improving the quality of care and management of patients with C. *difficile*, a bacterium that causes symptoms from diarrhea to life-threatening inflammation of the colon. Hota says, "That got me into stool transplants, or fecal microbiota transplantation, which is basically taking stool from a healthy donor and giving it to people who have intestinal illnesses. In fact, we're learning a lot of different health issues may be tied to your gut microbes. You're trying to replace them to improve or in some cases cure that problem."

It's a difficult question to phrase properly, but I ask her what it was that drew her to stool transplants. Hota says she liked the academic side: "Here's a treatment that needs to have a good study that's designed to evaluate how well it works, and it's simple, and I could see how this could change the way we approach treatment of this disease. And then, of course, there's the actual impact of the illness on people in hospitals and the whole health care system."

After C. *difficile*, Hota dealt with the emergence of H1N1 influenza in 2009, which she describes as the "pandemic everyone forgets." So she has already faced a broad range of challenges, from academic to administrative. But it was those times on stage, singing, that helped the self-described shy kid deal with Covid's media spotlight, including one of the most interesting moments: when she was being interviewed, in the early days of the pandemic, and the host was handed a piece of paper with some breaking news. Hota knew about a significant development in the Covid story that had not yet been made public. She sat in the studio, live, waiting to hear what question would come next and wondering how she would handle it. As we say in the news business, more on that later.

———

DR. FATIMA KAKKAR

Pediatric Infectious Diseases Physician
Clinician-Researcher, CHU Sainte-Justine
Associate Professor of Pediatrics, Université de Montréal

A BACHELOR OF ARTS DEGREE, WITH A MAJOR IN POLITICAL science, is not the typical path to become a doctor—and it did require a stint in summer school to catch up on a couple of required courses—but Fatima Kakkar recommends it enthusiastically: "I actually tell all my students, if you want to go into medicine, do whatever you want for your under-grad because it's such a time to learn about everything. You're going to learn medicine for the rest of your life."

For Kakkar, there was an additional incentive to get that BA. She says she entered university unsure what career she was headed to: medicine, law or international relations. Her parents moved from Afghanistan to Montreal in the late 1970s. Her dad, Gul Mohammed Kakkar, had lived there as a student in the late '60s, getting his master of law at McGill. He returned when he was posted—temporarily, the family thought—to work with the United Nations' International Civil Aviation Organization. But when the Soviets invaded Afghanistan in 1979, Gul and his wife, Nafisa, decided to stay in Canada and start a family.

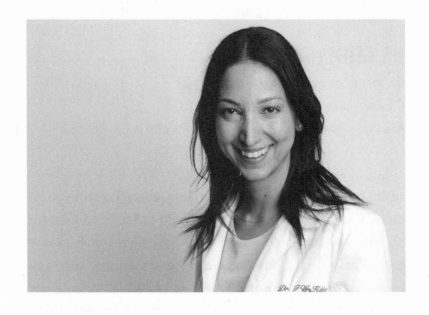

Dr. Fatima Kakkar, Montreal.
Photo courtesy of Dr. Fatima Kakkar

Because her father had come here as a diplomat, Fatima was able to go to an English-language school. And like so many first-generation immigrants in Montreal, the Kakkars glided between cultural groups. "So it was English at school, French with my friends and Persian with my family."

When I ask her about high school, she is enthusiastic and candid, describing herself as "a big talker. I ran the debate team. My friends were 'Change the world, save the world,'" she laughs. Her family travelled a lot, in part because of her father's job but also to see relatives. "I would spend summers in India and Pakistan and Iran, so being part of that big global picture was something I was interested in, and it was sort of my reality."

She went to a small all-girls school, Miss Edgar's and Miss Cramp's—yes, that is actually its name—where she had what she describes as "a great experience": "My family and I were very unique, so everyone wanted to know about our background. It was a lovely school where everyone was very open to my culture and my family."

As you would expect, she did well—"I was a good kid, very studious and got good grades"—but her focus went beyond academics. Kakkar was also a basketball star. "I'm very tall," she explains, matter-of-factly.

She says the school gave the students confidence that, as young women, they could, and were expected to, succeed and be in charge: "Girls were at the head of the table, girls were on the debate team, and I think that had a huge influence in giving me confidence and being able to speak in front of large crowds. They really put that at the forefront. It was a huge influence. We didn't see any barriers. It was only later in life I saw how things could have gone in a different direction."

Beyond the support of the school, she says the "anglo Montreal bubble" that she lived in felt very comfortable. "I didn't sense I was different, being an immigrant, having a different religion."

In Quebec, high school ends with Grade 11. University-bound students then go on to a two-year program at a public or private college. For Kakkar, that was Marianapolis College in Montreal. It was, she says, "day and night" from her small high school. "You do whatever you want, study whatever you want. There were not as many rules and so many more ethnicities. It's the first time I noticed people segregating into cultural groups—Southeast Asian group, Asian group, the old private-school group. We all had our little bubbles. I was with the all-private-school white girls. I didn't identify with my culture, there were so few Afghans."

Academically, Kakkar was unsure what career she wanted. She decided the easiest option was to do a general health sciences degree, but she also took law classes and sociology. After graduating, McGill seemed like the obvious next step.

But what she took there, that bachelor of arts, with a major in international relations, "came as a big shock to everyone, including my parents, who thought I was going into math, engineering, science, the doctor route." She loved what she studied—learning Arabic, for example—but also how she studied. "The science crowd is very much very methodical, there's a very set way to study for your exams and take notes, and you don't miss classes and you do every single reading and it's a very different crowd than the poli sci crowd. You sit, you talk, you write, it's all very informal."

But it was during a class lecture by the head of Médecins Sans Frontières that her career choice came clearly into focus. "We all wanted to change the world . . . but what skills will you bring to this? What skills? I needed a practical skill I could apply, so I decided I wanted to go into medicine."

So, once again, Kakkar took a turn that surprised people around her. "When I was asking my poli sci professors to write letters of recommendation, they were a little miffed. They asked me, 'Are you sure this is not for law school?'"

The letters—along with her marks and interview and MCAT test results—must have been supportive. She got into McGill's medical school. Except there was one small technicality. She didn't have two of the required courses, Organic Chemistry 1 and 2.

She had successfully completed the chemistry questions on the MCAT and thought perhaps her lack of two prerequisite courses had slipped under the radar. It hadn't, and Kakkar ended up taking them, concurrently, in summer school.

As much as she enjoyed her arts background, she is quick to concede it made first-year medical school more difficult. There are no courses in first year on the *British North America Act*. Instead, she was expected to know the fundamentals of biochemistry and physiology. "These are things the other med students had majored in, and it was tougher for me to keep up." Like a lot of medical students, she had those moments where she wondered if she was doing the right thing.

As she continued her studies, Kakkar says one of the most gratifying activities was spending time with the international students at the medical school. The young woman whose community at Marianapolis was "private-school white girls" was now becoming friends with students who had a connection to her family culture. "For the first time I got to know people from the Middle East, an Arab contingent and Persian contingent, people who grew up very similar to me, friends from all over the world, more similar to me than people I had met before. These people have become my lifelong friends."

After medical school, Kakkar did her residency in pediatrics at Western University in London, Ontario. "I love working with kids . . . they're fun and funny. It's a joy."

While at Western she worked on medical missions in Honduras and Africa. It was there, in Zambia in 2005, that she had an experience that left a deep impact.

She and two other pediatric residents from Western were working in the village of Monze. Kakkar says that, in Canadian hospitals, "to see a child die is so rare, and we don't have children dying for a lack of basic supplies or equipment." But in Monze they had one oxygen generator, and with that came choices no one should have to make.

"I had a child with end-stage HIV who was on the oxygen, and we had a baby come in who needed the oxygen. Do you take the oxygen from the child who is going to die within days to give it to the baby? It was heartbreaking. Here, in our hospitals, you go into every room where there is oxygen. You open the valve and it comes out. It's flowing. And to not have basic oxygen was more than eye-opening. It highlighted the magnitude of the problems and also how privileged we were here. The three of us, when we got back, we were pretty shocked when we came back to our regular hospital work."

That experience guided her to infectious diseases, not only to continue to work in global health but also to concentrate on HIV research.

"I always knew I wanted to do something international. I wanted to go to Africa and back to Afghanistan. I wanted to work in global health, and I needed more than a general pediatric degree to deal with HIV, malaria and TB."

She did her fellowship in ID in Toronto and then went on to a sub-specialty in HIV. It was through her HIV work that she reconnected with Alex Wong, whom she had worked with during training in Windsor, and who she would see at conferences in Canada. Those conferences, of course, stopped during the pandemic. But it was the pandemic that brought them together again, virtually, in February 2021.

———————————

DR. SRINIVAS MURTHY

Pediatric Critical Care and Infectious Diseases, BC Children's
   Hospital
University of British Columbia

IT IS WELL INTO OUR INTERVIEW WHEN SRINIVAS MURTHY mentions, almost in passing, how his experience during Ebola outbreaks prepared him for the early days of the Covid pandemic. "Ebola?" I ask him. Only then does he tell me about being sent to Liberia in the middle of the Ebola outbreak of 2014. He had been doing consulting work with the World Health Organization, travelling to work on diphtheria and measles outbreaks. His dual specialties—critical care and infectious diseases—and his research into pandemic-prone infections and hemorrhagic fevers led to a months-long assignment to West Africa.

The US Centers for Disease Control describes Ebola Virus Disease as a "severe and often deadly" disease that spreads through contact with the blood or body fluids of infected animals or humans. Among the symptoms are abdominal pain, vomiting and bleeding. I tell Murthy that Ebola sounds terrifying to non-medical people like me, and he assures me it is terrifying for doctors too. "You are worried that you are going to get it, much more than, say, I worry about getting Covid. And the life in the community, despite it not being as transmissible a disease as Covid, because of the individual fear of the disease, your life is very different. Limited contact with individuals, streets were reasonably empty. You go to the store for bare necessities only and then you go back home. While I knew, because of my privilege, I would be evacuated if I got the disease, still I knew it would not be pleasant to get infected."

Murthy led Liberia's national case-management response as well as treating patients and training doctors. By the time of Covid, he was familiar with responding to an epidemic. "You can plan for an emergency, but there's nothing like the experience of living through it, the structures that need to be in place, how you make decisions.

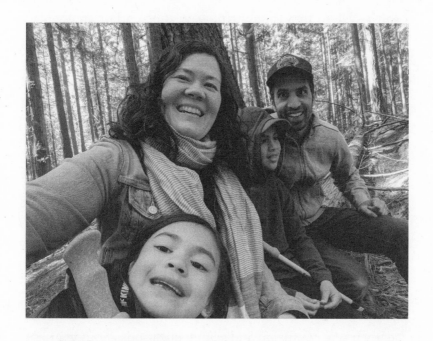

Dr. Srinivas Murthy with his partner
and children in North Vancouver.
Photo courtesy of Dr. Srinivas Murthy

"Sadly, a lot of the experience of the last year and a half in North America, a lot of the world has had that, responding to a severe outbreak and being able to coordinate a health system in a thoughtful way. Those other emergency responses in health care, that experience is obviously very useful when you're applying it to Covid."

Dealing with infectious diseases like Ebola, diphtheria and measles around the world were formative experiences for a young doctor a long way from home.

Murthy was born in St John's, Newfoundland and Labrador, the youngest of three children. His father, Gummuluru Satyanarayana, and mother, Bala, had emigrated from South India so his dad could do post-doctoral work at Memorial University.

Murthy says that being of Indian descent in St John's in the '80s and '90s was, to his classmates, "a unique concept." He explains, "It's not that racism didn't necessarily exist, but mostly it was confusion and asking questions about your life kind of thing. It came less from a place of malice and more a place of not knowing, and you got to educate them about your culture and where you came from. A great place to grow up."

I ask him to describe the teenage Srinivas: "I think he was awkward and shy and wanted to see what the rest of the world was like. Like most teenagers, you had your pluses and minuses." And like everyone in this book, he doesn't mention his academic achievement until I bring it up, saying he must have been very good at school. "Yeah, I think so. I won awards in school and at science fairs and math competitions, junior high and high school. And in undergrad. School was not a major hurdle for me."

Interestingly, for someone who clearly would have had his choice of undergraduate schools, and who describes himself as someone who wanted to see the world, he didn't go very far for his first degree: Memorial, his hometown university. He says, "[It] was more from a practical perspective, like money and a lot of my friends from high school were going there. When you look back at my high school [grad class], I think only five or six kids went to universities outside of Newfoundland."

He excelled at science but also minored in philosophy, which he said was exciting to study and read. By "mid-undergrad," though, he was pretty sure he'd be a doctor. "It may have partly been being a child of Indians, being in medicine was a default in a way." It was a path one of his older sisters had already followed.

Finally, at age twenty-two, Murthy moved away to go to McGill. He had been to Quebec for French immersion and grew to love Montreal. I ask him what stood out about his medical school years: "A lot of my work in med school, at least the first few years, was focused on a lot of advocacy and activism. This was at the time of the HIV pandemic, and access to medication, primarily in sub-Saharan Africa, was a challenge, getting medication to the right place."

He sees parallels now with access to Covid vaccines: "Exactly the same issue, coming again. So seeing that pandemic in medical school set me up for this one."

HIV medications were expensive, and many people in poorer countries couldn't get access and were dying. "That sort of injustice was pretty motivating. Particularly at that time, there was a lot of advocacy on trade negotiations, and I became very well versed in how patents were protected and so on. I testified in Parliament in second year of medical school on this exact subject, trying to advocate for Canada specifically and more globally for medication to be available to folks in poorer countries." Murthy's activism was motivated, in part, by his friends. "If there were evenings and your options are should we just go and hang out at the bar or should we work on this proposal or project together, if there are people you like who have common ideas, that's what you do. And those people remain friends to this day."

When he applied for residency, the next step after medical school, he says he eventually hoped to do both infectious diseases and critical care. He liked "the clinical management" of very sick patients as well as what he describes as "the beauty of infectious diseases."

I ask him what that means. "When you think about human history and the way we interact with the environment around us, and what causes diseases and has the largest impact on human health, infectious diseases have always been at the forefront of that relationship, whether it's TB or malaria or plague or what have you. Our environment has shaped us, and will continue to shape us, both in health and disease, and this makes for hugely interesting thought processes."

The kid from St John's continued to see the world, doing his residency in Harvard and then heading to Toronto for his infectious diseases fellowship.

"To travel around for training I recommend for all my trainees . . . no one place does it completely right, whatever 'it' is."

After moving from St John's to Montreal, Boston and Toronto for training, Murthy is now in Vancouver for work, and, pre-pandemic, was travelling to various hotspots around the world. Which brings us back to Ebola in Liberia. Murthy admits it was, in a certain way, exciting. "I'm a critical care doc and I thrive on adrenaline to a certain extent, and there's nothing more adrenaline inducing than being at the centre of the world's largest outbreak."

But the enormity of the task was never far from his mind. And while he knew, if things got too dangerous, he had the option of leaving, he watched as "local doctors were dying in huge numbers because of a lack of protection and a lack of equipment." He gained an insight that a lot of front line workers around the world have likely thought about during this pandemic. Murthy asked the Liberian doctors why they kept volunteering. "They said, when you're called on by your society and you have a skill set, it's your duty to offer that skill, and we are the warriors of our people. And this is our time to fight."

DR. LYNORA SAXINGER

Infectious Diseases Physician
Medical Lead, Antimicrobial Stewardship, and co-chair
   COVID-19 Scientific Advisory Group, Alberta
   Health Services
Associate Professor, University of Alberta

DYSTOPIAN LITERATURE VS. MICROBIAL GENETICS. WITH AN unusual academic flip of the coin, Lynora Saxinger decided she would let her final mark in those two courses determine what she'd choose as her undergraduate major. It came down to a single percentage point. Microbial 92, Dystopian 91. The winner, by the slimmest of margins, microbiology. So perhaps it won't surprise you to hear Saxinger describe her younger self as, among other things, "quirky."

She grew up in Saskatoon. Her mother, Bernice, was a registered nurse, and her dad, Walter, who came to Canada from Germany, was a tailor, though Saxinger says, "In another lifetime, if his mom hadn't decided he had to be a tailor—because that was a trade and she was parcelling out to the kids different trades—I think he would have been a really good engineer."

In high school she was "the kid who hung out in the arts room. I felt it was a personal failing if I didn't get extremely good marks, but I was very quiet about it. I was a little bit goth-emo in personality and tendency rather than preppy or jock, which were the only other options when I was growing up." She says she doesn't remember a lot about high school, but when I ask her to give me a little more detail about what she was like then, she pauses for a long time and says, "I was . . . just a bit . . . alternative. Alternative music. Alternative clothes. Liked to read a lot. Liked doing art. But held myself to a high standard on science."

For university, she stayed in her hometown and says studying microbiology was "fun." She spent one summer doing genetic research on—what else—"bovine herpes viruses" at the veterinary college laboratory. That came with the very vet school perk of "having lunch on the lawn with a baby yak and a ferret," which were housed at the school.

She figured the next step was to get a master's degree in microbiology, but "I had a lot of pre-med applicants in my class, and it hadn't really crossed my mind to apply for medicine until I was, like, 'I'm smarter than that guy, he's applying to medicine, should I apply to medicine?'" she tells me, laughing.

When it came to her transcript, however, Saxinger had what you could call an arts disadvantage: it was hard to get the grades required for medical school in literary criticism and studio arts classes. But she did get on the waiting list, and then: "I got in, and I thought, 'Oh dear, do I actually want to do that?'"

She remembers feeling a little intimidated when she walked into class on the first day. "I was wearing Doc Martens and cut-off men's trousers and a black turtleneck. So, kinda dressed up." She laughs. "I looked around and thought, 'Do I belong here?'"

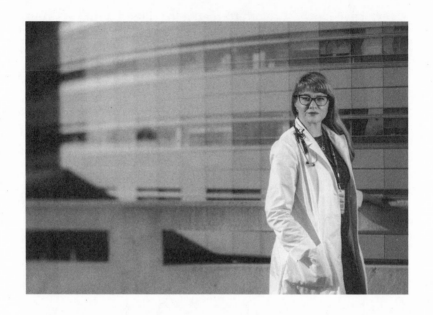

Dr. Lynora Saxinger, Edmonton.
Photo by John Ulan/UlanPhoto.com

It didn't take her long to feel more comfortable in that class, eventually becoming president of the Student Medical Society, among other things. With just seventy-five students in her class, she says the University of Saskatchewan was a "fantastic place to train. You do everything directly. I did tubal ligation, bedside liver biopsy, You were working directly with the staff. It really was an excellent place."

Medical school was "an interesting experience in letting you figure out what your strengths and weaknesses are and, if you have strengths, maximizing it." She laughs. "It is very much that 'Be all you can be' Army slogan thing. I quite enjoyed it except for the horrible parts, and appreciated the experience. It's a huge responsibility to become a physician, and it's also a privilege. People trust you and you can do high-impact things."

After graduating, Saxinger moved to Edmonton for her fellowship in internal medicine. She says this allowed her to delay her decision on what to specialize in. "I'm plagued by being interested in a lot of things, honestly." She chuckles. "I think people who can form a focal interest and excel in that one area do better." She considered other sub-specialties, but "because I had the background in microbiology in undergrad, I kind of always knew I'd end up in infectious diseases, although I tire-kicked a lot of other things on the way."

She also made a couple of stops that had a formative influence on her as a physician and a person. The first was spending three months in Zimbabwe in 2001.

She says, "It was still in the midst of difficult times in terms of the AIDS epidemic, with essentially no HIV therapy available in the country, and limited therapies for other things we could treat there."

There were riots, political unrest, and people in the hospital went a month or two without being paid. But most difficult, she says, was watching patients die because there just weren't the resources to deal with them. "[It was] so hard to accept there were things I could see and diagnose but I couldn't treat. I would admit twenty-five patients a night, which is a lot for an internal medicine service, and we would have so many deaths every single week, of things I would have been able to treat if we had been in Canada. It was just heartbreaking."

Sometimes they would send families to pharmacies to try to get the medicines their relatives needed. Too often, those patients died, their bodies stored in refrigerated trucks at the hospital until the families could find the money to pay the hospital bills.

Saxinger says there were excellent local doctors, "and I remember thinking, 'How can they keep doing this day after day?' because I know I was feeling morally distressed at the end of the first two weeks. I figured out what they were doing was looking at things and thinking, 'I can't help that, I can't help that, I CAN help that person.' They tried really hard to do the thing they could do and then they kept on. That was how they were managing to keep going. Once I figured that out, I was able to have a more productive time there."

She points out, "It's also an incredibly beautiful country, which I completely adored. It wasn't all bad, but it was a vivid experience in many ways. I worked at a leprosy unit, a multi-resistant TB unit. I had to bike everywhere because there were petrol shortages. It was a very important experience for anyone who's interested in health care."

Another formative experience came in a much different setting, as a visiting physician in Boston. Saxinger joined the ID team at Massachusetts General Hospital, home of the *New England Journal of Medicine*. "All of the staff people had published in infectious diseases, so I was a little star-struck." She was also hit by a feeling lots of Canadians—perhaps especially those from smaller places—might find familiar.

"I was thinking, 'I'm this girl from Saskatchewan and I'm working with all these Harvard medical students.' I was prepared to be intimidated. Instead, I think the biggest thing for me, besides seeing some really interesting clinical cases, is what I learned is a good medical student in Harvard is as good as a good student in Saskatchewan. The difference is at Harvard, they're all like that. It's not a different scale. It's just the concentration. I felt very happy I was holding my own and I was contributing. It made me feel less worried about coming from a small medical school and a place no one had heard of."

Still, she felt some people wondered just how rugged and exotic her home province was. "I think they were surprised I walked upright," she jokes. "It was kind of fun because I was able to surprise them frequently if I knew what I was talking about." She decided to play to the stereotypes when she presented a case she knew of a patient who got botulism from eating muktuk in the Canadian North. "I thought let's just run with this," she says, laughing.

"They're going to come away thinking I live in an igloo but what the heck."

There is no igloo in the Saxinger family history, but she does say her dad and uncles hunted, and the family "ate deer and moose fairly regularly." Saxinger says she has no interest in hunting, but she does like shooting and is perhaps the only person in this book who has taken a rifle marksmanship course. "As it turns out, I'm a pretty good shot. Still won't be shooting anything living—but target shooting is very fun. The people at the range are pretty interesting to listen to."

The young woman who wondered if she belonged in medical school has now been an infectious disease doctor in Alberta for twenty years, training a new generation of students. She tells them, "When I'm on call for infectious diseases, it's like guest-starring in people's nightmares for a week." And it's clear from her tone, and what she says next, this is not a glib description. "It could be the worst thing that happens in their entire life. And you're the consultant and you're coming in and talking to them about it. And you have to be careful with that responsibility.

"If I'm seeing patients in clinic, there's a wait-list to see a specialist. They might be coming from out of town and staying in a hotel overnight. I have to be on my game. It's a very significant event for them, where for me it's a string of events. But I am really drawn to high-impact work. I get a lot of internal value and motivation from that."

Saxinger says, "I'm struck again and again at how resilient people are and how sometimes people, for example, who have addiction problems and injection drug use and complications from that, are amazing survivors and often incredible people. The one I'm thinking of specifically was a young woman who had been in hospital two or three different times with heart valve infections from injection drug use, and she was very young. And I said to her, 'When you're using injection drugs, can you go over your technique with me? Maybe we can talk about ways to prevent infection.' She's telling me what she does and I say, 'Why do you do that?' And she said, 'That's what my mom and dad do.' I thought, 'Whoa, you never had a chance. Your mom and dad taught you how to use injection drugs. That's not a great start in life.' But she was really, really smart and really, really capable. Obviously a true survivor. I think that realization is important when you're looking after people, to have an open mind when dealing with everybody."

For all the doctors in this book, their approach to the pandemic draws on their experiences with patients, their expertise in infectious diseases and, to an extent, their personality. For Saxinger, "I've always gravitated to practical, complex problems. By practical, I mean when you see something you think someone should do something about, or something that seems like it could be better, that's always something I've found it easier to engage with than more purely arcane, academic, scientific pursuits. I like to question dogma. I like figuring things out. I enjoy that." She pauses before delivering the punchline. "So I'm kind of like the most at risk for Covid-obsessed-behaviour person that I could imagine."

DR. ALEXANDER WONG

Infectious Diseases Physician, Saskatchewan Health Authority
Associate Professor, University of Saskatchewan

WHEN YOU'RE LITERALLY NAMED AFTER A HOSPITAL, IT would be easy to say you were destined to be a doctor. And yes, Alex Wong says his mom always wanted that for her son. But there was a time when he didn't think that was going to happen and was assuming he would end up in a completely different career.

Wong was born in Edmonton at—wait for it—the Royal Alexandra, where his mother, Emily, was an ICU nurse. She "provided me with the health care background. It was a very stereotypical Asian household. High expectations, very idealistic, teaching hard work and focusing on what you can control."

His father, Chi, completed his post-doctoral work at the University of Alberta, and the family moved to Scarborough, Ontario, when he got a job as a chemist. Alex's extremely self-effacing description of his teenage years? "I would have been the mega-nerd who had no fashion sense whatsoever. Hyper-competitive, reasonably athletic for someone with Asian genes and no height. That's why I got into racquet sports because I couldn't do anything else. I was actually on the basketball team for a couple of years. Then I stopped growing."

Just in case your picture is not vivid enough, Wong adds, "I was on the frickin' math team. I did the Reach for the Top stuff, all the quintessential nerd stuff, but at the same time I had a hyper-competitive streak. I think if you were to ask anyone who knew me, that's what they would say. I think the word 'intense' comes up a lot when people think about me. I learned over time to temper that intensity in ways that were productive and to realize maybe there are times when you need to shelve that a little.

"I probably didn't grow up and figure things out from a social perspective until my early thirties. And that's helped me with my perspective as I deal with marginalized and vulnerable people who have far less privilege than I do."

Wong said the academic part of school came easy to him, but the first couple of years of undergrad "were a bit of a struggle" when, like so many students, he was figuring out how to navigate the new-found autonomy. His major areas of study were biochemistry and computer science, which, for a future doctor, seem fairly reasonable, but he laughingly describes it now as "a combination of mega-nerd type things. On the spectrum from cool to completely lame, I would be very close to completely lame." Still, he points out, "Everyone grows and matures in your own way. The traits I care most about are, I try to do the right thing—my dad instilled that in me. I care about integrity and saying what I mean and following through and doing what I say I'm going to do and having consistency that way."

Wong's path from undergrad to medical school should provide comfort to anyone who has been discouraged while trying to take a big step. He says he applied three times and sat on wait-lists at various schools. He started thinking seriously about an alternative career and was interested in becoming an educator, either at the public school or university level.

But while working at a summer job on the Scarborough campus of University of Toronto, he got the call. He'd been accepted into medical school at Western University in London, Ontario, and remembers how momentous that was, thinking to himself, "Wow, there you go. My life has changed."

When I ask him about his time in med school, he says it was probably "pretty comparable" to everyone else's experience, but he does point to his third year, when Western began offering medical students the option to move to Windsor. Wong took that opportunity, and it had a big impact on his training.

"It was nice to be in a place where you had a lot more autonomy and a lot more independence as a student. There was less competition for the attention of mentors, and we had access to the best teachers because there was a real desire on the part of the medical community to make everything work. Mark Awuku, a pediatrician, Raphael Cheung, Dale Ziter, these are some of the people I am still in touch with to this day and are extraordinary physicians and great mentors."

The first time I spoke to Wong was on *The National* early in 2021, when he was on a panel alongside Fatima Kakkar. As it turns out, "Fatima and I met each other for the first time when we were in Windsor, and Mark Awuku, who's one of the best pediatricians in the country, was the main teaching physician there at that time. Fatima and I had worked together briefly—now we know each other because we're

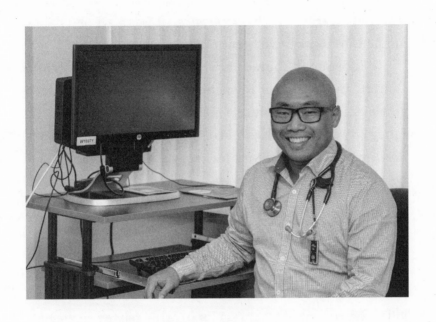

Dr. Alexander Wong, Regina.
Photo courtesy of Saskatchewan Health Authority

infectious disease people—but right after that *National* spiel I texted Mark with the link, and I gave him a call, and we had a nice conversation to reminisce about what he taught us as medical students and first-year residents, now we were featured together on *The National*, so it was a bit of a happy moment to think back to our training."

Windsor, of course, is right across the river from Detroit, and Wong got to spend time in that city. "The biggest piece that stood out to me when I visited some of the inner-city hospitals like Detroit Receiving, you could see how much greater the issues around socio-economic vulnerability and challenges were compared to Windsor. There was a much larger divide between have and have-not populations in Detroit."

What he saw there would have an impact on his practice years later. "It very much is this traditional inner city with racialized populations, African American, Hispanic, and a lot of chaos, a lot of trauma, a lot of other related challenges, and then you go out to suburbia, massive houses, mansions. It is the sort of typical divide that exists in the United States, and it gave me a bit of a flavour of the challenges that exist within the system."

Wong went to Edmonton for his internal medicine residency, where, he says, "The chief residents of our program, the people who were leading the residency program as peers, they all said, 'We're doing infectious diseases.' So I thought to myself, 'Well, if all of these smart people, who seem like they have really good hearts, are choosing to do infectious diseases, they must know something about it, right?'"

Infectious diseases appeals to what Wong says is a basic part of his personality: "I'm the sort of person who likes the concepts of social justice and advocating for marginalized, vulnerable populations. I chose internal medicine because I'm a Type A, micromanaging person who likes to be thorough, and to me that fits what it took to be a good internal medicine doctor. I chose infectious disease fairly early for a variety of reasons. The ability to advocate for social justice and to help advocate and work with populations that don't necessarily have a voice was definitely a huge part."

That Type A personality trait certainly played out when he began to search for a place to practice, he says, and he did locums across the country, from Moncton to London, Ontario, to Regina, before deciding to settle in Saskatchewan. "It really appealed to me. It was similar to Edmonton in terms of marginalized, vulnerable populations, a large proportion of Indigenous heritage, a lot of social chaos, a lot of inequality.

"One of the main reasons I chose to come here was because there was a huge HIV epidemic, and that's driven by many complicated dynamics: colonialism, residential schools, historical trauma, all of these pieces which are extremely impactful. And you can talk about some of the other stuff which is a little more tangible, our opioid crisis, the overdose crisis, but it stems from inequality."

Wong concedes, "I didn't really understand how complex and intricate those issues were probably up until two or three years ago, when I made a concerted effort to begin to try to enhance my own understanding of history, as well as making a decision to move into trying to help people with a variety of addiction-related issues. It's something that goes hand in hand with what a lot of infectious doctors do, what we deal with in our hospitals, in our clinics and what we do in a longitudinal basis with blood-borne infections like HIV, viral hepatitis, specifically hepatitis C. And in the hospital we see a lot of people with infections on their skin, bloodstream infections, many infections related to addictions or mental health challenges."

To better understand the context, he took "formal coursework on the history of residential schools, the history of some of the cultural genocide that's taken place. Understanding what culture-informed and trauma-informed care looks like, and getting formal training and mentorship on addiction training as well. That has become a significant part of my day-to-day practice now, and it allows me to provide more holistic care for people I see in the hospital and clinical setting."

Wong says that in his ten years on the prairies he's learned a lot about how to effectively advocate for what he calls meaningful change. "Everybody's got different interests, different focuses. I'd like to give everyone the benefit of the doubt and say everyone wants the best possible outcome. Sometimes you need to take a little time and energy and try to understand what everybody's perspectives are, and what people's priorities are, and find ways to bring people together.

"I didn't quite have that understanding before. I was much more bang your fist on the table, 'what's wrong with you, how come you can't see these obvious things, how can you let people die?!' I realized quite quickly that even though that approach and messaging sometimes feels like it will make a difference in the moment, it's not usually the most effective way to really get to where you need to get to."

That change in approach was about to be tested in March 2020 when a colleague sent him mathematical modelling on potential Covid spread, and Wong realized he needed to convey a sense of urgency to public health officials.

CHAPTER 3

TOP OF THE ROLLER COASTER

THINK BACK TO DECEMBER 31, 2019. THE LAST NEW YEAR'S Eve before the pandemic. Many of us were out at dinners and parties celebrating the promise and optimism of 2020.

Infectious disease doctors remember that day for something else: a notice from ProMED Mail, a service of the International Society for Infectious Diseases that reports ID outbreaks around the world. It was posted at one minute to midnight, December 30, with the title:

Undiagnosed Pneumonia—China (Hubei):
Request for Information

What followed were sixteen stark sentences. Very little information from a place most of us had never heard of. Here's an excerpt:

The so-called unexplained pneumonia cases refer to
the following 4 cases of pneumonia that cannot be

diagnosed at the same time: fever (greater than or
equal to 38c); imaging characteristics of pneumonia
or acute respiratory distress syndrome; reduced or
normal white blood cells in the early stages of onset.
The number of lymphocytes was reduced. After treat-
ment with antibiotics for 3 to 5 days, the condition did
not improve significantly.

It is understood that the 1st patient with
unexplained pneumonia that appeared in Wuhan this
time came from Wuhan South China Seafood Market.

Patients with unexplained pneumonia have done
a good job of isolation and treatment, which does
not prevent other patients from going to the medical
institution for medical treatment. Wuhan has the best
virus research institution in the country, and the virus
detection results will be released to the public as soon
as they are found.

Susy Hota says it was enough to raise concerns: "You get a ton of those alerts. Every day there are a few that come through. Most of them are nothing, but that one definitely caught my attention, and I definitely got that feeling. We know THE event can happen, a pandemic can happen. An unknown severe respiratory illness cluster coming out of China is sort of the prototypical event that you're looking for. The uneasiness never left me after that. It was that discomfort that started snowballing."

Lynora Saxinger also remembers the email well, though she says she might not have looked at it closely until New

Year's Day. "I don't always read my ProMED mail," she laughs. "It might be about tomato viruses or whatever." But she too realized this one was different. "I remember reading about a mysterious pneumonia in China . . . and I went, oh dear. It made me think of avian flu and pandemic, and I remember thinking, 'I wonder what that will be. It obviously has an association with SARS . . .'"

With so little detail but so much concern, Srinivas Murthy was soon emailing colleagues in different parts of the world. "This was just when we were seeing reports from the seafood market, before we even knew that human-to-human transmission had occurred. It was still in Wuhan. They hadn't panicked. Case counts hadn't spiked yet."

Still, the alert stood out. "Even then there was a large degree of anxiety about what we were hearing. Did I know at that time it would produce everything that ended up happening? No. But we all had spidey senses that this was different from all the other reports we'd heard about over the last few years."

You may remember some of those "other reports." A bird flu from Asia, for example, which caused a flurry of concern and coverage in Canada in 2008 and then seemed to go away. Murthy said those earlier infections always turned out to have "predictable transmission patterns, predictable severities." By contrast, an "unknown pneumonia" outside a seafood market in a crowded region of China had the potential to be significantly different. "I think all of those features combined enough to make those of us who paid attention to it at the time a bit more suspicious."

Isaac Bogoch was on a brief vacation when the email came in. He says his in-laws were visiting and taking care of the kids, so he and his wife headed to New York City. But it didn't turn into exactly the trip they'd planned. With a laugh he says his wife "was annoyed with me because I was on the phone a lot of the time, talking to my friends and colleagues, saying, 'Whoa, what is this? Is this the real deal? Is this SARS Part Two?' because SARS One had a similar appearance. This really was a small red flag at the time, but it needed careful attention. And of course I watched it like a hawk over the next couple of days to see more data that emerged from Wuhan, and we heard more and more people were infected."

Like his colleagues, Bogoch points out how little information was available outside China in those first few hours. "No one knew that it was a coronavirus. People weren't even sure it was transmissible from human to human. No one knew what the source was, but it was clear this problem was bigger than initially advertised, and what we started doing immediately, we came up with the idea January 1, we need to look at this further."

"We" was a group of doctors that Bogoch had worked with before, mapping where Zika, a virus that can cause severe birth defects, and Ebola would likely spread based on travel patterns. With the World Health Organization set to meet in mid-January, he and his colleagues analyzed information on the potential spread of this new virus. "We wanted to collect useful data to drive sound policy . . . make policy based on high-quality data."

Bogoch says the team started to look at travel patterns from Wuhan to the rest of the world. They submitted their findings to the *Journal of Travel Medicine*, which quickly reviewed the work, sent some revisions and then posted it online on January 14, just over two weeks after the ProMED Mail alert.

A paragraph in the journal article, which is titled "Pneumonia of Unknown Aetiology in Wuhan, China: Potential for International Spread via Commercial Air Travel," captures both the concern and the uncertainty:

> *Seventeen years after the global SARS epidemic,*
> *the current outbreak in Wuhan, China serves as a*
> *reminder of how rapidly novel pathogens can appear*
> *and spread with potentially serious global conse-*
> *quences. Although it is unclear what the current*
> *burden of disease is or the potential for human-to-*
> *human transmission, major Asian hubs are the most*
> *probable sites of exportation should this epidemic con-*
> *tinue, and public health officials are already on alert*
> *in those locations.*

At this point, whatever was happening in faraway Wuhan was having no impact in Canada, other than getting the attention of a number of doctors. We were still going to work, crowding into subways and onto planes. Lynora Saxinger says the story "almost went underground for a while, and then it started percolating again." Once in a while a piece of news would stand out. Saxinger recalls, "The next thing that really struck me is when they built the hospital in China in ten days, which is pretty impressive. But at that point it still seemed quite remote, and, to be honest, sometimes it seemed like science fiction, quite removed from our lives."

And then there was Italy. After the first reported case in late January, infections soared, prompting a lockdown of more than fifty thousand people on February 22. Soon we heard the harrowing, heartbreaking stories of hospitals overrun with sick and dying patients. According to the *European Respiratory Journal*, more than 190 doctors and nurses died in Italy after being infected with Covid. Among the likely reasons, according to the journal, was a shortage of personal protective equipment (PPE) and a lack of proper ventilation in hospitals, but also "doctors were working under extreme pressure for many hours without any breaks or days off, probably decreasing their attention towards protection." And as they got sick, it put more pressure on those who were still working.

Murthy says, "When Italy was having its 'everything falling apart moment' was when the ICU and outbreak community [in Canada] realized this was something really bad. The initial Wuhan experience could have been attributed to poor planning or that it got really out of hand really quickly. Then we saw they managed to reduce their case counts." Other countries, Murthy pointed out, like South Korea and Singapore and Thailand, "seemed to do a good job containing outbreaks with good public health and good infrastructure."

Italy felt different. Murthy says Covid cases "started to fill up every hospital in their region and had hundreds and hundreds of deaths within days, I think that was our 'Come to Jesus moment,' so to speak. This is going to be a big big deal."

As it turns out, Murthy was in southern France at a World Health Organization meeting as the Italian outbreak surged out of control. "There was a lot of anxiety. There were no cases in France at the time, but it was just across the border, and we had to drive to the airport across an Italian hill or something like that, and everyone was suspicious. 'Are we safe here? What's going on? It's over there, but is it over here?'"

Susy Hota says the tempo of calls and meetings among hospital infection control departments quickened. "We were constantly in communication, my colleagues and I in Toronto and also broader groups. 'When do we need to advocate more or escalate something?' And we realized we just weren't doing enough surveillance to know when we would get into trouble in Toronto, in Ontario."

Hota recalls, "I think there was a lot of discomfort in the early part of February that we weren't doing enough to pick up infections. We knew it was coming and we don't want to pick it up at a point where there's so much ongoing community retransmission that you can't get a handle on it. That was a disturbing time for sure."

By the end of February, confirmed cases in Canada were still so rare they were being reported one by one. And while the identities of patients were not disclosed, some details were being made public. On Thursday, February 20, there was a news conference in BC about the case of a woman in her sixties, the eighth positive test in the province. What made this one different was she had travelled from Iran.

Bogoch says that was extremely troubling. "A very astute clinician in Vancouver did a Covid test and it was positive. That raised a huge red flag. If a country is exporting Covid cases, the burden of infection in that country is probably a lot larger than what's being reported." He's quick to clarify. "I'm not pointing fingers. A lot of places don't have the capacity to report for a variety of different reasons." But he says that one infected traveller landing in Canada was likely a sign of "a bigger, hidden problem."

With two colleagues, Bogoch "reverse-engineered it and looked at travel patterns and flights and volumes of passengers from Iran globally and from Iran to Canada. Using the probability of a person getting infected and landing on a flight in Canada, that would suggest you have a significant burden of infection in Iran that's not being reported or not being identified." The analysis, "Estimation of Coronavirus Disease 2019 (COVID-19) Burden and Potential for International Dissemination of Infection from Iran," was published in the *Annals of Internal Medicine*.

Bogoch says the Covid-infected traveller from Iran was "one of the soul-crushing parts of the pandemic, because once Iran was a huge hotspot for infection it was clear this was not going to be contained. Iran was one of the sentinel events. It told us this is very very widespread and there are probably a lot of other places that have a lot of infections that are not being identified and not being reported for a variety of reasons, and we're going to have ourselves a pretty nasty pandemic."

Here's how the journal article described it:

> The lack of identified COVID-19 cases in countries with far closer travel ties to Iran suggests that cases in these countries are probably being missed rather than being truly absent. This is concerning, both for public health in Iran itself and because of the high likelihood for outward dissemination of the disease to neighboring countries with lower capacity to respond to infectious disease epidemics. Supporting capacity for public health initiatives in the region is urgently needed.

As dire—and prophetic—as that sounds, remember what life was like in Canada in February and early March. Many people were getting ready to head south for school break. University campuses were filled with thousands of students going to class and partying. The NHL and NBA were still playing to packed houses. We were shaking hands, hugging friends and sharing equipment at the gym.

In Edmonton, in February, Lynora Saxinger says, "There had been a feeling of invincibility because we were across the ocean from [Europe and Asia], which is ridiculous, and even at that point there was already some spread in the US that wasn't detected. But there was a sense this was someone else's problem, and that continued for some time." Saxinger pauses and adds, "I think we should all collectively reflect on that process where the countries that have been used to dealing with influenza strains that could be pandemic strains, they were right at the epicentre of this pandemic, and they saw it way better than everyone else."

That sense of invincibility was being felt in many places in Canada. In Montreal, Fatima Kakkar says, "We didn't think it was going to be as major an issue as it turned out to be. I'll be honest, January and February, in Quebec, we were overconfident. We had a smattering of cases. I didn't actually think it was going to be as serious as it was—and then people went on March break."

Like British Columbia, Quebec also had a case from Iran in late February that raised alarm, at least for the medical community. Kakkar says there was a debate: "The ministry would only let us test travellers from China, and we were arguing about this case from Iran, which had been detected by mistake. We said, 'Let's screen everybody,' but the answer was 'No, follow guidelines, we don't have enough tests.' I remember thinking at the time, 'We're missing the boat.'"

By March, the agonizing hospital stories from Italy were being echoed in New York City, with social media posts describing the constant wail of sirens, overcrowded wards and exhausted health care workers. On the West Coast, Washington State was in the midst of a full-blown Covid crisis, but thousands of people were still driving back and forth across the border with British Columbia each day. And BC—and the rest of Canada, for that matter—seemed relatively untouched in those first days of March. That, of course, was about to change.

For most of us, the turning point came in the second week. The World Health Organization declared COVID-19 a global pandemic on Wednesday, March 11. That night the NBA suspended its season. As all this was happening, even the experts were trying to figure out how it would affect them and their communities.

The week before, Lisa Barrett had been at two conferences, one in Montreal, the other in Toronto, and neither about anything remotely connected to Covid.

She was asked to do an interview for CTV, and the producer brought up the growing number of Covid cases. "I hadn't been paying attention for a couple of days, and when I heard the rising numbers I thought, 'Uh-oh.'" I ask her, more than a year later, what she recalls about that interview. "I remember saying there was no reason to panic at this point. Whatever happens, we're going to stay on top of it."

Then she returned to Halifax and "walked into our boardroom that we were going to use for the next nine months as a situation room, and it feels like we never left."

Barrett says a colleague had looked at the number of people infected in China and some other places, and the percentage who needed hospitalization and admission to ICUs, and applied that calculation for Nova Scotia. Barrett says it was a sobering moment: "This is the number in terms of deaths and hospitalizations, even for our own little province. We stopped and paused and said 'Wow.' And that was the start of a very different approach for all of us infectious disease docs."

Barrett says that instead of asking if anyone in the health system needed help and guidance, "we just said we're going to do what we're going to do. Building clinical trials, doing research, advocating and hopefully someone agrees with us and brings us along, because this is a problem and we've got expertise. I remember writing down, 'We need clinical trials here, we need to get drugs here or we're going to watch people die.'"

Other infectious disease doctors in other cities were having a similar experience. Saxinger remembers having "a distinct feeling we were staring at a train barrelling towards us, and we were just standing there blinking, and that was not the appropriate response."

In Regina, Alex Wong says, "It didn't probably get really real for me until about the third week of March, when it became readily obvious that we needed to move into a red alert situation. I can pinpoint the day. I work closely with a computer scientist in Saskatoon, Nate Osgood, a really smart guy. He was tasked to do the original modelling [on potential Covid spread] and was working on it basically since Wuhan came out. He put forward a devastating modelling presentation in the third week of March that basically predicted that we were going to get completely destroyed.

"I saw that presentation. I was sitting on my couch, he'd sent it to me. I read it and I just had this awful feeling: we are screwed. As it turns out, that didn't happen, and that didn't happen for a variety of different reasons, but it was one of the times I have felt that so-called pit in my stomach."

In a variation of a question sports reporters ask athletes about getting to the big leagues, I ask Zain Chagla what was his "welcome to the pandemic" moment. Turns out, quite appropriately, it was from the NBA. "I watch a lot of basketball—it's one of my favourite things to do in my free time." On March 11 he was in front of his TV as the tipoff for the Utah Jazz game kept being delayed.

"Utah is one of my favourite teams. [Jazz player] Rudy Gobert wasn't coming out, people were asking what was going on. Then we heard he'd tested positive, and another player tested positive, and literally within fifteen minutes the NBA suspended its season."

In the CBC newsroom in Vancouver, the NBA's news flashed across our computer screens, and I remember how many of us (and yes, we were still crowded at our desks) looked at each other, stunned. In the newsroom we quickly turned on an NHL game in Edmonton, where the Oilers were playing the visiting Winnipeg Jets. It was unfolding, with thousands of fans and workers (including, by the way, one of my sons), as if everything was fine. But we started wondering if this would be the last NHL game for a while.

It's strange now to think how a professional basketball game in the United States brought home to so many of us that this global pandemic was about to have a big impact on our lives in North America. Turns out it was the same for at least some infectious disease experts.

Chagla was sitting on his couch in Mississauga. "It was just like, 'Oh God, this is real. This is the first major institution [in North America] that was affected by this.' I had Raptors tickets the next week. I was supposed to take my cousin, and I remember texting the week before saying, 'I don't know if we're ending up going to this game or if it's going to shut down or go into some minimal crowd capacity.' But when that NBA game stopped, that was a moment that the world had changed. We had seen lockdown in Italy at that time, and looked at it and thought, 'This is wild,' and then Wuhan locked down . . . that looks wild . . . Now, when the NBA shut down, you had the sense in the room this was coming really really soon, and yes, by two days later we essentially put our entire society into lockdown to deal with COVID-19."

Sumon Chakrabarti's "welcome to the pandemic" moment was the next day, Thursday the 12th. "I'll never forget this. I was driving home from tennis. The NBA had just shut down, and what I remember was the gas prices. Whatever it was, it dropped to seventy cents. It was one of those things where I wondered, 'What's going on here?' I turned on the radio and all they're talking about is the pandemic."

That weekend, more things started shutting down. We were told to be prepared to start working from home, and by Monday, Canada was a very different place.

For doctors responsible for infection control, one of the first significant impacts was the change in the number of meetings. Chagla says, "We went from a couple of meetings a week to a couple of meetings a day to essentially all-day meetings." He says the challenge was adjusting infection control plans from something theoretical, based on past experience, to something very real that they still didn't fully understand.

"We had planned for an Ebola case showing up in Hamilton or planned for a novel pathogen showing up, but as we saw this march from Wuhan, Italy, Iran to other places in the world, the meeting schedule started picking up, the time invested, the uncertainty, the surge planning, the infection control, personal protective equipment. All of that just started taking up time, and you start seeing the growth in time [devoted to Covid] and anxiety among patients and staff. As medical director it was hard trying to balance that while trying to be calm and follow the evidence when very little of it was actually coming out."

In March 2020 there was still little known about SARS-CoV-2 (short for "severe acute respiratory syndrome coronavirus 2"—the virus that causes COVID-19), and the experts were experiencing the same anxiety many of us in the general public were feeling. In Regina, Alex Wong says he had some sleepless nights. "I was sani-wiping my office literally on an hourly basis. I woke up in the middle of the night to wipe my car down because I was, like, what if there's SARS Covid 2 in my vehicle? I haven't cleaned my vehicle. And all the anxiety. I continued to take the kids to daycare, which remained open for essential workers, and it was just eerie. My kids were literally the only two kids in the entire daycare with a staff of seven."

At Regina General Hospital, Wong says there was deep concern. "We were right in that period where everything in the news was about the impact around the world. New York was being devastated. Northern Italy. Spain, Portugal. They had already been devastated.

"Everyone was scared and you could see it in everyone's eyes. It was quite something for me to see. People were wondering, 'Are we all going to get sick? Are we all going to die? Are we all going to bring it home to our families and our loved ones? What needs to be done here?'

"I approached the different unit managers and we set up some informal Q & A's. I would stand at the front of the ward, at the nursing station, and everyone gathered. I tried to provide people with some reassurance, with updates on what we knew about science, what we didn't know, what was appropriate and not appropriate. Do we need to shower? Do we change all our clothes? Do we need to bleach our groceries? Do we need to alcohol-swab the Tim Horton's cup before we drink out of it?"

For Fatima Kakkar, the end of March break stands out. "All of a sudden our Covid wards, our ICU wards, began to fill up. That was the trigger that this was not like SARS, this is way bigger. We had our protocols in place, and [in Infectious Diseases] we were working on what we were going to do. How are we going to isolate?"

At Sainte-Justine pediatric hospital, Kakkar says, "We had set up a Covid testing centre, and we were seeing many people come back with fever. We had lots of PPE, so we were head-to-toe PPE and thinking, 'Now this is real.'

"That same week the Jewish General Hospital, which is the Covid referral centre . . . Originally was going to be the only Covid centre, but within days the ICU filled up. The exponential increase in hospital admissions told us something was off."

Kakkar says it was an anxious time for her. "Everything shifted in the hospital. We were wearing masks everywhere in the hospital, distancing on wards. We in ID have the most bravado, we go see Ebola patients, we're not scared of anything, but that was the first week where at a physician level, and at a hospital level, this became real, it became serious."

Travel plans and conferences were cancelled. Kakkar says, "All of a sudden we were told, 'You're not leaving Quebec. This is going to become a medical emergency.' I remember the sense of worry. We'd seen the emails from the docs in Italy . . . That's when we knew it could get very scary here."

On April 1 the first pediatric patient was admitted to Kakkar's hospital. The mother was a long-term-care worker, the dad worked at a factory. The whole family tested positive. Kakkar says she thought, "This is the tip of the iceberg. I wondered how many people really were infected . . . and it occurred to me this is way bigger than we had thought it was."

As Isaac Bogoch thinks back to March and April 2020, he remembers the anxiety over the unknown. "We really didn't know enough about this virus to have a high degree of confidence as to how we should protect ourselves or how we would treat patients. We had some ideas, because it is an infection and we're in the business of treating and preventing infectious diseases, but there is a healthy fear of the unknown, or maybe a better way to frame it is a healthy respect of the unknown."

He remembers how eerie it felt stopping to fill his car with gas on the way to work in the early days of Ontario's lockdown. "It was very early in the morning, the streets are empty, businesses are closed. I'm the only person around at the gas station. I remember replacing the nozzle and thinking to myself, 'Is this a risk? Can I get this infection from this?' I had some hand sanitizer in the car, but it's that kind of thing that crossed my mind."

Walking into the hospital, Bogoch remembers, "You have your mask on, you've got your face shield on, your gown, walking into a room to see a patient, and, you know, I think I'm okay, but I'm not sure. It was unnerving, it really was. I'd go through these cognitive exercises and try to rationalize the healthy respect—and fear—of the unknown. We know this is a respiratory virus, we know how respiratory viruses are transmitted, and we know how to protect ourselves with appropriate protective equipment. And that really helped. You just go back to first principles and realize we're going to be okay."

To be an infectious doctor at this time meant people inside and outside the hospital were looking for guidance. Bogoch says, "I don't speak for everybody, but I know many of my colleagues in infectious diseases were getting phone calls from family, from friends and community organizations with questions we had some answers to, but we certainly didn't have all the answers at the time. There was a tremendous amount of anxiety in the hospital, throughout Canada, and globally at that time. And a lot of that anxiety was projected onto infectious disease specialists."

He pauses. "I've never gone through something like this in my life. This was really hitting us at home and it was very personal."

In Hamilton, Chagla was "seeing patients, and the meetings were six to eight hours a day. There was a huge amount of anxiety. We didn't know a lot about the virus. We have no treatment that was evidence based, vaccines aren't even on the table. So all of us were kind of sitting there saying, 'Well, how is this going to look in six months or a year? Is it going to rip through the population?'"

He recalls this is when the "flattening the curve" messaging started coming out. "It's almost the top-of-a-roller-coaster feeling, you know. You're looking down, you see this drop, you know it's going to be painful for the foreseeable future. It's that pit-of-your-stomach feeling. It's just coming and there's nothing you can do to avoid it at that point."

It was a blur of meetings, personal feelings and, of course, dealing with patients.

Complicating things, says Chagla, was that "colleagues and friends became patients. Thankfully they didn't have severe complications, but I followed them virtually or over the phone and gave advice. It was tough to see, obviously. It was definitely an eye-opening experience just seeing the spectrum of people who got it and how they dealt with it."

In Mississauga, Chakrabarti candidly admits that there were times in March when he "was waking up every morning with a sense of anxiety. Every single day—and I don't mind admitting this—I actually worried about dying."

His hospital started to implement its pandemic response and, he says, "I was thinking, 'I'm infectious diseases.' I was going to be on the front lines. And yes, initially I was afraid of what might happen. I remember telling my wife that."

He recalls walking into the rooms of the first couple of Covid patients. "I had my protective gear on but I was so nervous. I was standing far away from the person. But after seeing a couple of them I realized, 'Yes, they have a disease that's communicable, but I've seen hundreds of these in my career,' and we started to say, 'Look, we don't need to be wearing space suits to protect ourselves.'"

There were still nervous moments. "At the time, we weren't sure how much touching things was an issue, so I remember washing my hands like crazy, and one time I worried I hadn't washed them properly and I touched my mouth. Slowly those things settled down. We knew we were protected, and we could see everyone else was much more calm."

The anxiety of Covid might have been subsiding, but the emotional impact was about to hit hard. A friend of Chakrabarti's, Dr. Rick Singh Mann, posted a story on Facebook about the death of his father-in-law at Trillium Health Partners—Mississauga Hospital: "He died in the ICU at our hospital despite the amazing care he received from the exceptional nurses and doctors who looked after him. Despite being on a ventilator, COVID-19 took just seven days to take him away."

Dr. Mann's post, which was widely covered by the media, provides a poignant glimpse into what was happening at the hospital:

My wife and I are frontline health-care work-
ers, which makes this time especially challenging.
The night he was admitted, I had spent the day in
meetings at our hospital to create a triage zone for
COVID-19 patients. I spent the next three nights work-
ing overnight in the emergency department, screening
dozens of patients for COVID while also providing care
to our usual sick and wounded, meticulously applying
and removing protective equipment again and again
to help prevent the spread of infection.

We applied that same protection when we went
to see my father-in-law too. Every time. No touching,
no sitting in the room to comfort him, no long visits to
talk and reminisce. The risk of infecting ourselves, our
families and our patients was too high.

Shortly after my last overnight shift, he got
worse. We drove back to the hospital to talk about
his wishes for end-of-life care, and he was moved to
the ICU. The next day he was placed on a ventilator
because it was becoming impossible for him to breathe
on his own. Yesterday he expired.

Chakrabarti had gone to medical school with Rick's wife, Nooreen, who gave him permission to talk about her father's case. "Her dad had come back from a trip and he wasn't feeling well, and they wondered if they should get him tested. And then within seven or eight days he was admitted to hospital and, of course, got very ill and died. It was a wake-up call for all of us because, first of all, he was one of our first cases here in Trillium, and second of all, it's someone close to you. It has just that much more of an effect on you."

Still, Chakrabarti says even as the number of cases grew and they were dealing with the tragedy of Covid deaths, he started to feel a sense of confidence. "We saw how the disease manifested, saw we were not going to be Italy or New York City. I wasn't afraid of it anymore. Of course, I wasn't going to go in the rooms without PPE, but the actual fear of being in a room with patients and dying was now gone. A sense of duty had taken over."

Wong agrees. "Yes, we were on the front lines. Yes, there was massive anxiety with regards to looking after patients with Covid, especially in the times when we had no idea about how to protect ourselves, what was risky, what was not, what was transmissible, what was not. But I saw it as my duty. It's our duty to look after people who are sick. And you don't function well or at all in any meaningful way when you're scared. So trying to curb the fear and focus on being strong and confident for the patient is really important."

While careful not to identify the patient, Wong says he vividly remembers his first interaction with a Covid-positive person. "I had a resident with me and I had a medical student with me and I said, 'You're not going to go in there. I'm going to be the one who goes in there.'

"The patient was not that sick," Wong continues. "He had recently returned from travel, and other than me providing reassurance, the majority of the time was spent with him begging me for hydroxychloroquine, which was the medication at the time that was being touted as a possible treatment, and we spent half an hour going back and forth about the pros and cons.

"I was doing my best to focus on his questions. I was keeping distance. I was standing at the foot of the bed, probably about one or two feet away from the foot of the bed, so well over six feet from him, and I had the whole kit and kaboodle on in terms of PPE, N95 [mask] and all the rest of it all, and I didn't feel that vulnerable. I felt like it was important—even though I was kind of scared on the inside—I just had to do the right thing and project confidence and not fear because people would look to me, and if I'm scared, if I'm not sure, I'm trying to avoid patients with Covid, that's not going to set a good example for anyone else."

In Vancouver, as in many cities across North America, seven o'clock became a symphony of clanging pots and pans in appreciation of front line health care workers. I remember walking by Vancouver General Hospital, worried about what was happening inside. Srinivas Murthy says, "The original BC experience was relatively mild. We had our first death in March in a long-term-care facility, and the hospitals were never overwhelmed. We never had the experience of New York or Lombardy or Wuhan in terms of the system strain. We had patients but it was within the flow of things, and we had planned accordingly to expand ICU and hospital capacity, hopefully in a thoughtful way."

I ask him if it was frightening. "It's always frightening when something new is happening. I would say I myself wasn't frightened that I would be severely affected because of the data I had looked at and my risk profile, but also I had been in a number of Ebola and influenza outbreaks around the world. If you know how to deal with that, you feel more confident, despite not knowing everything about the pathogen. You can use your personal protective equipment and knowledge and risk assessment to get through it the right way."

At a more systemic level, he says the lessons Canada learned in the last year were lessons many other places in the world had already lived through. And having been through some of those crises helped him prepare for this one.

"Having an experience with emergency response . . . Everyone does simulations, everyone has an idea as to how people would respond or how you would respond in an emergency and how your governance structure would work and who would make decisions. But none of it is a replacement for experience. Every simulation, every piece of paper you write, falls apart with details. So having experience with emergency response to emerging infections obviously had a ton of value in this context."

And so, across the country, infectious disease doctors continued to have meetings. Lots of meetings. People were brought together to figure out what was happening and what should happen next. Lisa Barrett remembers the challenges in how different people took different approaches to decision making. She said for some people "there's a lot of pride in being right, and some people have trouble backtracking. I think one of the characteristics of our group as a whole— and I think it served us pretty well—is that we're okay with making decisions . . . and okay, we'll change it if we need to.

Some people think there's a risk you'll look silly, but there's no ego to the group. It was 'Okay, we may be wrong, but let's overreact for a few minutes.' Not panicking but a reaction that might have to be walked back."

As the sense of emergency deepened, one of the challenges, says Barrett, was who should be involved in influencing policy. I ask if she was part of the discussion about creating an Atlantic Bubble, which restricted people outside Atlantic Canada from entering the provinces of New Brunswick, Nova Scotia, Prince Edward Island and Newfoundland and Labrador. "Definitely not. I think all provinces struggled to get the right people in the room for those sorts of conversations. I think the P [politics], E [economics] and the V [virus] were not always in the same room. I think there was a fair bit of creating silos. Not everyone was in those groups all the time."

Eventually, Barrett says, it worked out. When I interview her in the spring of 2021, she says, "Now there's at least an infectious disease person at most of the tables. But still there are an awful lot of tables at the P, E level of things that make decisions."

For all the doctors, the workload increased, but the tasks were different. Susy Hota's main responsibility was dealing with infection control measures in hospitals. Describing it to me, she compares what she did to the usual role of public health officers, except within a more highly infectious environment. As the pandemic hit, "the workload became much denser, and longer days. There were twelve- to fourteen-hour days of tasks, meetings, and that could go through to the weekends. Some of it is building protocols, writing policies, engaging with different groups, providing education presentations, working with the executive team to overcome problems. I sit on a number of committees, national committees and provincial as well as regional."

One committee Hota sits on oversees hospitals in the Toronto region of Ontario Health. She's the infection prevention and control lead, and she says, "This is where we develop our hospital policies on things like universal masking—people wearing masks in hospitals at all times, which never existed before this—all the screening that happens at the door. So it's putting the policies into action and making sure the right measures are in place, it's going to be feasible and take into account the human factors of it. So a lot of what I do is not your typical infectious diseases."

Many of the other doctors were dealing with those "typical" infectious disease tasks, except in the highly charged atmosphere of a quickly changing pandemic. And they realized they would sometimes have to take on new roles.

Wong says when his colleague showed him the modelling, which predicted Covid infections could potentially overwhelm the Saskatchewan hospital system, he wanted to make sure public health officials in Saskatchewan were fully aware of the dire projections. He says he asked his colleague, "'How confident are you in regards to all of this?' and he was, 'Yeah, we are super confident.' We've collaborated on other research, on other projects. I know how smart the guy is, and I was, like, 'We are in massive trouble here. And we need policy makers and decision makers to understand with complete clarity what needs to be done ASAP.'

"So he and I ended up working with the internal modelling group with the health authority, and we basically put together some very focused presentations for our chief medical health officer, focusing on the really key measures, which obviously were distancing and public health restrictions combined with testing and tracing. So the need to aggressively ramp up our testing capacity as quickly as possible, and ramp up our public health test and trace, and isolate to keep from crashing and burning, and that was essentially the simply message that Nate and I and others within the modelling team realized we needed our policy makers to hear and push as quickly as possible."

In the province to the west, Lynora Saxinger says the biggest demand for her time in those early days of the pandemic came from Alberta's Scientific Advisory Group, which she co-chaired. She says there weren't a lot of Covid cases in the province at that point, and the advisory group became "the overwhelming focus of all my time." Its first report was published on April 4, and the title reflects both the priority at that point and the reliance on careful research: "What is the optimal strategy for healthcare worker [HCW] clothing and personal items across various health care settings to reduce the risk of HCW self-contamination and to reduce the risk of healthcare workers transmitting viruses outside the hospital?"

Three days later the advisory group released a second report that addressed two questions about the risks and benefits of oxygen therapy. In April alone, the advisory group posted seven reports, from analyzing which Covid patients need intubation to determining when it is safe to discharge patients from hospital.

In the first weeks of the pandemic, Saxinger says, "I probably spent way more hours with that group than anyone in my life." Like so many people in other fields, members of the advisory group were meeting virtually. Saxinger reflects that it was "a strange intimacy . . . we spent so much time together but never met in person." Their responsibility was to "funnel the immense churn of information for decision makers. Early on, the research and the meetings took sixty hours a week." And although the time commitment eased as summer approached, Saxinger says the Scientific Advisory Group remained "consuming, professionally."

It did come with at least one side benefit, at least for members of the public. When the media started calling, Saxinger says she realized she was able to answer questions because she was already well versed in the very latest Covid research. And across the country, those media calls kept coming.

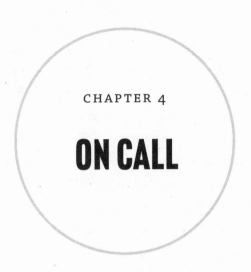

CHAPTER 4

ON CALL

I SOMETIMES FEEL LIKE I CAN'T ESCAPE ISAAC BOGOCH. That's a sentence I wouldn't have imagined writing pre-pandemic, and I realize even now it requires some explanation. Every Sunday, as I prepare for *Cross Country Checkup* in the CBC Vancouver studio, there he is on our news channel. On a Monday morning, as I walk into the gym, Global is streaming on one of the TV screens, and there's Dr. Bogoch. I see his name in a promo tweet for Peter Mansbridge's podcast. I see him on the CTV News Channel. CP24. And, of course, on *The National*.

Add the other eight infectious disease docs, in five time zones, and multiply it by all the outlets covering this story. In the first few weeks of the pandemic it seemed like there was at least one of the doctors on the screen every hour of every day. And beyond traditional TV, radio and newspapers, there is the dizzying array of other media. Zain Chagla and Sumon Chakrabarti appear on a fellow doctor's Facebook Live town hall, Lynora Saxinger chats with Ryan Jespersen for his independent multi-platform webcast in Edmonton, Fatima Kakkar is featured on a French-language podcast, Srinivas Murthy on an English-language Punjabi community radio station, Alex Wong talks to students via Twitter, Susy Hota is quoted on a University of Toronto news site, Lisa Barrett is interviewed in a video on SaltWire (and yes, I had to do a quick search to discover SaltWire is a website with news from across Atlantic Canada).

For months I wondered how the doctors kept finding the time. And perhaps more fundamentally, why they continued to say yes.

For Bogoch, "It just sort of happened. People kept calling, and I kept answering the phone. I'd done media before—for example, with the Ebola epidemic in West Africa and with Zika virus, the big outbreak in South America—so there were a few health reporters who had my number and email, and I'd been chatting with them early on in January about COVID-19. But, of course, the phone calls became more frequent. I tried to not let it interfere with my work and obviously with my life, but it's an important part of the job. I think that communicating to the general public is obviously extremely important, and I do my best."

Bogoch continues to do lots of interviews, but "it got to the point where you just can't accommodate all the requests that were coming in, and even today I unfortunately have to decline most media appearances. I really truly try my best to work with the media and accommodate as much as I can, but many of us have significant clinical responsibilities. I work at a university hospital, so there are teaching responsibilities and research responsibilities, and of course, with the pandemic, I'm on several different provincial or federal task forces that also require a ton of attention. So nowadays I really try to accommodate media requests for the early morning and for the later afternoon, and during the day I just put my head down and work."

When I spoke to him for this book, as the third wave was building in April 2021, Bogoch said he was averaging about three or four media interviews a day, done mainly in the morning between six thirty and nine, though sometimes he would squeeze one in during the day or, for *The National*, around seven in the evening.

During one of my conversations with Alex Wong, he mentions Bogoch with a combination of wonder and admiration. "The fact that he's continued to be this media presence, not just for CBC but pretty much every single news outlet, is extraordinary. I don't know how he does it. I struggle to figure out how to manage what I do. It's remarkable, right? He has been consistently solid, and there's no question that his only motivation for doing this is to provide good science and to provide clarity and a calming presence to the public."

As I explained earlier, being interviewed by the media almost always takes longer than you'd think. There are the technical requirements of making sure the audio and video are as good as possible. Everyone in the control room and studio has to be ready to go. And sometimes, with the goal of making the hit exactly ninety seconds—or whatever time is allotted by the program—there's a request to do it again.

So even with only three or four interviews a day, that's a big time commitment. But, again, Bogoch shrugs it off. "If you imagine a pie chart of how I spend my time, it's only a small sliver that's with the media. Dedicated time, it's probably a couple of hours a day when I add it all up. But most time is really with patient care or," he laughs, "in various painful committee meetings, task force meetings, that suck up a ton of time. And even between those meetings there's a lot of work that needs to be done in terms of preparation and outreach and whatnot. Most of my time is probably spent doing clinical care or on various task forces at the provincial or federal level."

And then there's family time, which has been another of this pandemic's challenges. "I basically spend every moment during the day either with patients or on a computer or on my phone, but I carve out time for my family too. I'm not always successful, but something better be very important to get into that five to eight o'clock time slot. Every day I try to—my kids are nine and seven—I try to prioritize family dinner every single night. It doesn't have to be fancy-schmancy, but let's just sit down at the table and chat, spend time helping with homework and spend time playing outside and jumping on the bed and reading with them. As abnormal and bizarre as this pandemic has been, there are some aspects that I'm trying to keep normal. I'm certainly not perfect, and there are days when that doesn't happen, but it does happen more days than not."

Susy Hota was also getting lots of media calls in January 2020, and, like Bogoch, she was almost always willing to say yes. "It was anybody. Any news outlet that had questions where I could accommodate. You feel a sense of obligation to help inform the public with what information you do have." And it was a wide range of public she was informing "Anything from local news outlets to national to, occasionally, international. There were some radio shows in the early days out of the US that were interested in getting a bit of a Canadian perspective."

Hota always has seemed so comfortable fielding questions that I was surprised to learn how shy she is. "Media does not come naturally for me. I do feel uncomfortable, but sometimes you need to go outside your comfort zone, and that can be a good place to be."

From a CBC News Network interview on a Saturday afternoon to blocking off ninety minutes on a Sunday for *Cross Country Checkup*, Hota is willing to let us encroach on her weekends. But, like Bogoch, she says it's not a big deal. Working on the weekends has long been part of her routine. "As an academic physician, we're kind of used to, unfortunately, working throughout the day, throughout the week, at nights. In my current job, it's very administrative, I have a lot of meetings packed into my schedule. I lead a department so I have HR things, a lot of issues to deal with, and I have my own academic interests, which are currently on hold. But before the pandemic there were many times I'd be writing manuscripts or having to do my research on weekends or after hours, and in many ways these activities have replaced that.

"I do think the workload in academic medicine is way too heavy now for everybody, and something's got to give.

And the pandemic has definitely stressed all of us and added to the variety of roles we've been playing in health care. But where it's possible to balance the time, I do. I work out almost every night. I see my kids, I spend time with them. Could it be better for each of these things? It's a work in progress. So I try to do my best to balance it all, including this."

Lynora Saxinger has also been a *Checkup* guest, answering questions and interacting with callers for ninety minutes on a Sunday. I ask her why she is willing to give us some of her weekend time. Here's part of her reply: "First, a thoughtful conversation is a rare pleasure, honestly, and if it wasn't kind of pleasant, I'm not sure even my pathologically overgrown sense of responsibility (also a factor) would always win. The pandemic has been lonely and isolating to everyone to some degree, and being able to connect a bit can be really . . . nice. We are all pretty invested in the pandemic survival experience, and sharing can be cathartic. And I really hope that answering questions as I can helps people. A variety of voices and ways of sharing information seems useful, as people likely value different types of communicators.

"Also, I think the right questions help me process all of the papers and data I'm looking at through a lens of what really matters to people—it's easy to get very granular scientifically, but then reframing as 'what makes a difference to people's lives?' helps prioritize."

As for her other media appearances, Saxinger thinks they started in February 2020, when the *Diamond Princess* became a big story. The cruise ship was docked in Yokohama,

Japan, with 2,666 passengers when there was an outbreak of Covid on board. Eventually almost 700 passengers tested positive. This was a huge story, so it's not surprising the media would be reaching out to experts for comment. It's also not surprising that, more than a year later, she can't be sure it was her first Covid-related interview. "It's all blurred together. Maybe it was before that."

As for her motivation: "I remember thinking, 'I'm getting more media requests. There's obviously a need for people to help contextualize information.' People were reaching out for that, and I think everyone in the media was probably having the same experience: whatever you usually did, you did now with Covid. So there were people with varying degrees of comfort with the subject matter, and there was a tremendous vacuum of information to fill. I was really worried because my perception was that vacuum was getting filled with BS, essentially. There was such a rapid spread of bad takes and bad information, and I was profoundly worried about it because at that time all we really had was public health measures [to slow the spread of Covid], so misinformation seemed to be a larger threat—still is actually—and the way it was playing out really worried me."

Saxinger says besides giving the public the most accurate information about Covid spread in those early weeks, she also was thinking about what tone she should have. "People were starting to get nervous, and I think the general feeling among [health officials in Canada] was 'Stay calm, we don't know if it's going to spread any further.' People were saying it's kind of like influenza. That was our paradigm for pandemic spread. In retrospect, we all kind of had our heads in the sand.

"I myself was quite anxious and watching what was going on. It still felt very remote to me, but at the same time I didn't think it was something we should be promoting widespread panic about. So there was a little internal tension there. You want to be honest but you don't want to be alarmist, and it was really figuring out where on that scale . . ." She pauses and then chuckles. "And that kind of scale has remained in the background throughout the entire pandemic."

Like Saxinger, Zain Chagla recalls that his first Covid media interview was about the *Diamond Princess*. But where Saxinger was on a traditional media outlet—a local Edmonton TV station—Chagla's interview reflects how diverse media have become in Canada. He says it was on "a web-based TV station from the Niagara area. It was a friend who had referred me to someone who was the director." Soon after, the demands started escalating. The PR department at St Joseph's Healthcare in Hamilton, where Chagla works, "started tapping me and my colleagues to do some more media. That was late February. It almost became a regular part of lifestyle around the time of lockdown."

We all have a sense of medical specialists being busy, but I want to get a picture of what busy looks like. I ask Chagla to give me a sense of how his schedule looked in 2020, even without the media commitments. He's the medical director of infection control at St Joseph's and was filling in at another hospital on a maternity-leave contract that turned into a full-time contract. Then, pre-pandemic, he took a third contract as a consultant at a hospital in Woodstock, Ontario. "I knew the manager there and she said, 'This is just a couple of hours a month, you just have to go to a couple of meetings and read a couple of reports and give some advice,' and I thought, 'Sure, that sounds fine.' But then, in the pandemic, it became very different for those three hospitals in terms of pandemic planning, dealing with outbreaks, PPE, integrating guidance from the province, communicating with medical staff, dealing with executive staff, which took up, probably, the vast majority of my time for the first three to four months, as well as working on provincial guidelines and developing local guidelines for treatment.

"And that's just the non-clinical standpoint. Obviously I still had my own patients, new referrals, some with Covid, some with other diseases, and people being scared, and questions, and the media stuff just started emerging in March.

"And there's research. In March and April I was involved in some ongoing clinical trials to get patients experimental therapy to make sure we weren't using things with patients that weren't actually working. That's an ethical paradigm that some people didn't necessarily follow, but for our institution we prioritized the epidemiology and testing, and strategies for personal protective equipment, and then lots of presentations, lots of stakeholder groups. A lot of people we were dealing with were scared."

In his description, Chagla didn't even include his teaching responsibilities at McMaster's medical school, where he's an associate professor.

Interviews with the media came on top of that. In the spring of 2021, he tells me, "It averages out to two or three calls a day, so twenty a week, twenty-five a week. Some of it's small, a clip for a newspaper article or an email, but some of it is intensive media. And then there's the writing. I think we've put out fifteen or sixteen op-eds over the course of the pandemic, and that takes more time than anything else."

Chagla says that he tries to do media interviews in the evening, "when there are fewer clinical demands and my schedule is more predictable. On days when I'm not on call, then I will try to slip in things over lunch or around three or four o'clock when the meetings die down.

"Anyone who reaches out mediawise, I've been pretty okay with chatting with. The more I do media, the more I realize different people watch different channels, and if it's important to reach out with a calm and evidence-based message, you have to be able to reach out to all channels in that sense. There are a lot of asks, and I've been trying to fill the ones I can fill without interrupting the more pressing stuff from a clinical and hospital standpoint."

Sumon Chakrabarti remembers his first Covid interview, in January 2020, on CTV. He says when Bogoch started getting more and more media calls, he referred some of them to Chakrabarti, who was happy to help. "I like this, I want to do this." Part of his motivation as the pandemic continued was to try to change what he was hearing in the Covid conversation, which he felt was both inaccurate and unhelpful.

"There's been a lot of stress on the bad news, a lot of stress on what we did wrong and a lot of blame as opposed to being transparent about what actually was happening and how we could change it. I've tried to be one of those voices in the news to make sure people know, yeah, this sucks, but it's not going to be like this forever.

"I want to help get the message across. I've always been very interested in medical communication. I'm by no means the smartest guy out there. Zain, Isaac, these guys blow me out of the water with their intellect, but one thing I think I'm good at is communicating difficult medical processes and concepts to patients or the public. I do a lot of communication at the hospital with people who are worried about the vaccine. I've been hired to help with that sort of stuff."

Chakrabarti says he thinks a lot about how to make his message clear. "Some of the other doctors have a research background and know the data, the trials, all of this inside out. I may not know that nearly as well as they do, but I do know the bottom line and what is important for the public. And that goes back to my love of distilling messages in a way the public can understand.

"I have a lot of friends who have been messed up badly by this pandemic—out of busines, depressed, drugs, alcohol, suicide attempts. I think when they're hearing bad news over and over again, it can become a weight. I try to talk about what's happening now and talk about what we're looking forward to in the next little bit. It's not being inaccurate, but framing it in a way to help them understand this too shall pass."

Some subjects have become so contentious that Chakrabarti is wary of talking about them to the media. "Certain topics have been especially politicized, and schools is one of them. If I have a request and the entire thing is about school questions, I just refuse. You say something and people attack you. People get really really mad at me."

But while he'll say no to an interview that's solely on a topic like schools, he will still answer a question about it in a more broadly focused interview. "I know it's important to a lot of people, so on schools I would say generally it's not a major driver of transmission unless you have a huge burden [of infection] in the community, and then I'd leave it at that. And talk about something else."

In our interviews on TV and radio, including answering live questions from listeners, Chakrabarti never seems to shy away from any topic. In fact, he says, "If there's something I don't know about, I can read it quickly, understand and communicate that. And I'm not afraid to say I don't know." He jokes, "I have said that I let my ignorance be my shield."

Chakrabarti is one of the many doctors based in the Toronto area who became prominent during the pandemic. In fact, four of the nine doctors in this book work in the Greater Toronto area. Partly that's because it is the most populous region in Canada and has the most hospitals and doctors. It's also where English-language TV networks are headquartered, so when experts were expected to come down to the studio, it was easier to focus on people in Toronto.

But the pandemic changed that. Not only did we start doing all interviews remotely—making it as easy to connect with a doctor in Regina as one in downtown Toronto—but the spread of Covid and the response of provincial authorities were different across the country. Local media organizations needed to hear from doctors who knew what was happening in their region, and national media needed that perspective as well.

In Halifax, Lisa Barrett figures that, pre-pandemic, she probably did no more than ten interviews a year, for print, digital and TV media. The topic was usually hepatitis C or HIV. By contrast, in the first twelve months of the pandemic she estimates she did about five hundred interviews, half of which have been for regional media. "Across Atlantic Canada," Barrett tells me, "I can't think of a news program or podcast I haven't done."

I ask her what approach she takes for interviews. "To be honest, I have tried to be appropriately opinionated. Often there's not a right answer in a pandemic, as information moves in Pandemic Standard Time. There's an interpretation, and I hope that people hear what I'm saying on that particular day and come back to see the next day and the next day, and feel there's more to learn."

In Vancouver, Barrett's fellow Newfoundlander Srinivas Murthy was also getting more calls from the media early in 2020 than he ever had before, "by orders of magnitude." He was familiar with the process, primarily from speaking about Ebola in 2014 when he was in Africa. Murthy thinks his first Covid interviews were with CBC TV in Vancouver. As I mentioned earlier, I do remember seeing him in our newsroom, back when guests were still dropping in. He also was doing interviews—in English—with the Punjabi media as part of his "outreach to the South Asian community" in British Columbia.

I wasn't sure how Murthy felt about doing interviews, so I was pleased to find out that he considers it "fun." Still, he says, "It's a lot of work, a lot of emails, 'can you spare five minutes here or ten minutes here.' In February, March [of 2020], it was all novel and fun, 'Yeah, hey, I can do that.' And people actually wanted to hear what I had to say, rather than [just] my family or people who work with me, which was nice, and I thought, 'Yes, I'll take it.' Then it got tiring after a few weeks and months as more and more things came in, so I deliberately said no to most people as I got busy."

Beyond identifying the doctors as infectious disease specialists, we often—at least on *The National*—add the hospital or university they work at. But Murthy says that complicated things for him. He tells me, "There was some institutional stuff. Speaking freely, depending on who you work for, is sometimes frowned on, so there was some going back and forth deciding who I could speak on behalf of, and what I could say, and that started becoming annoying and pushed me away from speaking to the media for a while. In the past few months [spring of 2021] I've been much more selective who I speak to and what I talk about."

That meant viewers didn't see Murthy as often as the pandemic went on. In contrast, you probably didn't see Fatima Kakkar in the first months of the pandemic unless you were watching French-language media from Quebec. Though she does her research and academic work in English, French is her primary language at Sainte-Justine, the Montreal children's hospital.

Kakkar says the number of requests from the communications department at the hospital increased when MIS-C (multi-system inflammatory syndrome) began appearing in children. "I remember I was on call during those weeks in April and, literally, we didn't know what this was, having patients with fevers who were going into shock, and we had no association to Covid at the time. We thought, 'This is weird. We're seeing all these non-infectious fevers,' and this was the month of April.

"And I do remember on Twitter, my friends in the UK were talking about seeing similar types of things, and that's how it all started. Then they came out with their initial findings and we knew there was this syndrome. The first interviews were based on that, and it was the French newspapers and French networks."

Kakkar was suddenly doing five to ten interviews a day, often with people she had never dealt with before. "Sometimes I had no idea who I was talking to. Afterwards I would find out it was this national podcast or newspaper. I was clueless." She laughs.

Her media experiences are an interesting insight into the unique features of Quebec culture. Kakkar quickly discovered the Covid story was developing differently on French networks. She needed to watch more of the coverage and began subscribing to the Quebec news channel LCN, Le Canal Nouvelles. "There were moments when you were in the clinic and the premier was talking, and sometimes he said things in press conferences before any of the physicians or public health people knew, so you really had to be plugged in to the French media to know what was going on.

"It was important to be able to pick up on the nuances of what [Premier] Legault and [Director of Public Health] Arruda were saying. The English components of their press conferences are really not the same because there is so much nuance in how they're saying things, and the details, so I felt obliged to really pay attention to the French media."

Kakkar says that, in general, the interview styles are different too. "As far as the questions, the French media is—how do I put this?—they're very direct. Much more direct. They're not 'gotcha' questions, but they do want to look at some of the controversies. So a lot about Quebec politics."

For Kakkar, a pediatric infectious disease specialist, many of the questions were about schools and whether the Quebec government was doing the right thing to keep students safe from Covid. The interviews were focused "much more on policy. There is medical expertise but a lot of policy."

She found the French-language interviews were also a little more freewheeling. "As far as question lines in the English media, you guys tend to pre-interview, go over topics. Not the same with the French media. It was a very different experience, actually, working with guys on the English side than the French side."

And Kakkar says it was clear to her that what she said in those French interviews, every word, was scrutinized. "It is a little tougher on the French side because everybody watches it within the hospital and the ministry of health. So you didn't want to say the wrong thing. Because the people on the committees, your colleagues, the people making decisions, may potentially be offended by what you're saying, or you may make the hospital look bad. It was much more stressful with the French interviews not to say the wrong thing, even though you actually want to say what you think. It was much more of a challenge to say what I think without worrying what the downstream consequences would be than, to be honest, with the English media. So few people within my hospital and, really, the ministry of health are listening [to the English media] that it's much easier to speak directly without having to think about a filter for certain things."

Besides the scrutiny she felt in her French-language interviews, there were also differences in how the issues were being discussed. "It becomes very political between the francophone side and the anglophone side because, from the get-go, the Quebec pediatric society said we have to keep schools open. The benefits outweigh the risks. Though there may be limited transmission, they didn't want to have masks in schools. There was a big outcry, and even Legault said it was because the anglophones were watching CNN and they were getting paranoid. There was a lot of anglophone media trying to prove schools were a source of outbreaks, which they weren't. So it did become political in that sense. The francophone versus the anglophone take on school reopening."

While Kakkar was navigating the unique politics of Quebec, Lisa Barrett was dealing with being a prominent voice in a small province. I know Halifax well—I went to university there and worked in the city as a television reporter. I tell Barrett that I assume the provincial government was very aware of what she was saying in her many media appearances. With her knowing laugh, she agrees. "Yes. Oh yeah. I think they watch the local news outlets fairly closely. You know, most of the time I get informal feedback. There's been a couple of times when you'll get an email or a text from some folks who will say, 'Hey, just wonderin' what you're thinkin'." But Barrett makes this very clear: "I have never gotten the feeling, nor have I been asked—and I'm being very frank—I've never been asked to temper or change my messages, nor have I ever been asked to deliver a message. I've never felt [the feedback] was an invasive thing."

Despite the scrutiny, Barrett has never hesitated to accept the media requests. Her reasons echo what I heard from all the doctors. "I do it because I do believe there's a need, and if you don't fill needs with good information, it gets filled with other things. People fill things with quasi-truths that really really are bothersome, and that's the main reason I do this. I don't think I have any power per se, but I do think a fair chunk of folks in the region at least pay reasonable attention, and," she quips, "that does give me chest pain on occasion.

"You don't want to be grossly wrong, but I can't be grossly wrong because I try to stick fairly closely to facts. And I'm also fairly transparent that we only know what we know today, and facts, so to speak, are likely to change as we get new knowledge."

While she's comfortable providing those facts, Barrett is reluctant to assess public policy. "If people ask me if I think a certain group is doing something in the right direction, I might comment, but I'm much more likely to say 'this is scientifically what is the right answer.'"

When I ask for an example of that, she cites government plans to reopen after lockdowns. "I'm perfectly comfortable saying, 'Here are the components of a reopening plan that make sense scientifically from an infectious disease perspective: Make sure you know the quantitative numbers. Make sure there's no community spread. Make sure your 'r' value [the measure of Covid transmission] is below this and you've got a rolling seven-day total that's going down.' That sort of thing. When I add, when pushed on occasion, 'If you do this, for example, solely based on dates and not other things, that's a little outside my comfort zone,' I do think it's important for people like me to say it sometimes. But that's the edge of my comfort zone because that's interpretational."

While Barrett, like most of the infectious disease doctors, began her Covid media experience by responding to a call, Alex Wong's first appearance came about because he made a call, reaching out to the CBC Radio morning show in Regina. He tunes in to the show each morning as he drives to work. One day in late March 2020, he listened to an interview and became increasingly concerned about the way a guest was answering some of host Stefani Langenegger's Covid questions.

"It felt kind of uncomfortable, listening to the responses," Wong says. "I didn't feel it was clear enough or the science was right. To be fair, there were so many unknowns at that point. So a huge part of this was trying to explain risks and benefits to people in simple, easy-to-understand ways, but also trying to be practical about it and safe about it as well."

Wong started doing one-hour question-and-answer sessions once a week. "I was trying to speak in plain, simple ways, not using scientific terms, or if one would come out, trying to make some effort to explain that, and having this comfortable back and forth with Stefani. I remember the very first one, I asked her to stop calling me Dr. Wong and start calling me Alex. A lot of interviews I did before Covid times were a lot more formal on a very specific topic, and you kind of prepare things and it becomes a bit more rigid than you would like. These Q & A sessions were very organic, it was almost like doing a podcast, where you had more freedom to explain things, as opposed to a TV spot, where it has to be very very focused and you have a couple of minutes and you're trying to get what you want to say in as concise a manner as possible."

Of course, being able to answer those questions requires you stay on top of the ever-changing information on Covid. Wong says he uses his evenings to keep up to date on the research. "It's a lot of work to stay current on anything, but it's even more work to stay current on Covid, where there's so much happening all at once. By no means do I know every last detail of every last thing that's happening with COVID-19, but that's my focus right now, given limited time, limited resources and a wife who hasn't left me yet but is thinking about it—and I say that in jest, but we've had moments where it's, like, 'What the, what are you doing? Why did you choose to take all this on?'"

Wong says he's settled into a late-evening routine. "Once the kids fall asleep, my wife and I will spend some time together, usually watch *The National* on YouTube, and then I'll go downstairs and I'll work from about nine thirty to eleven thirty. What I usually do is to collate all this information. I only follow a small group of individuals right now who disseminate really high-quality data and do it in accurate, concise ways. I'll review the data and review the papers, and then I put it back out on my Twitter account, and it almost acts as an editing exercise. That way, when I put it out there, it doesn't matter if anyone sees it, but it's more so that I've gone through the intellectual exercise of interpreting the data, trying to understand what the pros and cons are and how we utilize this data. It's like taking notes that I'm doing in a very public way on Twitter.

"When I post something, I'm pretty Type A. That's another things about ID docs. We're mega Type A micromanaging type folks. It's just the nature of infectious disease. And so this is the academic exercise I do, pretty much on a daily basis, so that if I get asked to do something, like if CBC News Network calls and they want to do a Q & A session today, then I'll probably be able to, off the cuff, answer questions and know it's accurate and I'm reasonably informed on what's going on.

"It does take time. My colleagues and I probably all have a morbid fear about not being prepared. Again, if we get asked questions where we don't know the answers, I personally feel very comfortable saying, on live television, 'I don't know the answer to that.' That is clearly the right thing to say."

Susy Hota knows what that's like. "Throughout the pandemic there have been countless situations where I've agreed to an interview, and I've been working my butt off all day and, lo and behold, there's been some breaking news and I just didn't really know about it. And I think that's one of the challenges of trying to communicate during a time of such rapid changes in what's happening. Quite often the experts you're trying to interview haven't had a chance to get to that information yet."

I ask her when she does her Covid research. "It is throughout the day. I don't earmark time to try to catch up on things. Some of my information I get from being on committees where we discuss what's happening, and periodically, in between things, I'm scanning what's happening in news. I scan Twitter at times, but that comes with a double-edged sword. It also sometimes gives me a sense of what people are talking about, among the five hundred things that have happened in the last twenty-four hours, what is really capturing attention. I do it before I go to bed, which is terrible for sleep. I do it first thing in the morning, with my phone. I hate that my children see that all the time. We were not a device kind of family before this at all. And yet that's what they see. It's very hypocritical and I don't like that, but it's the reality of what I have to do. I'm using multiple sources all the time."

When I ask Isaac Bogoch the same question—when does he keep up with the constant flow of Covid information?—it's the one brief moment when he seems, for about five seconds, slightly less than 100 per cent upbeat: "Ian, this sucks, it really does. I usually wake up at five thirty. Six is a good day. And I start my day by catching up on reading. I get the online table of contents from most medical journals that are relevant to me. I answer emails. I read the news and I'll start doing media, but I have my phone on me at all times, and it's sort of a constant stream of information coming in through emails or different channels to stay up to date, not just on the science and the medicine but also policy, because it's really interesting to see changing municipal and provincial and federal and international policy. It's a lot of work to stay up to date on what's happening around the world, and it's a lot of work to stay up to date on what's happening in Canada alone.

"It's not a dedicated time, there's no downtime. It's a steady stream of information through mainstream media, a little of it on social media, though I'm very skeptical about information on social media. And I got to tell you, I spend a ton of time on the phone, informally, with friends and colleagues in Canada and also elsewhere in the world, really listening. I really want to hear people's opinions and take advice. We can get stuck in our echo chambers very quickly, and I'm in a million different group chats. A lot of time I'm talking to people I know share a different opinion, and that's been very valuable. A lot of them are physicians or scientists. The other thing I've found very helpful is chatting with friends who are not medical or scientific, who are either in Ontario or outside, just to hear what they have to say about how things are going."

While Bogoch does most of his reading first thing in the morning, for Zain Chagla it's in the evening. He also says that while "social media has been a disaster for many reasons during COVID-19, one good thing has been the dissemination of information, of thoughtful discussions, or connecting with researchers around the world and seeing what's new with the evidence, how they're dealing with particular situations, having discussions around that. So that's after hours, and usually an hour a day—more when the pandemic was more uncertain, but now [April 2021] about an hour a day—keeping up on what's new in the literature and any new papers, therapeutic decisions, and really analyzing it as much as I can and looking at novel guidelines, whether or not we need to do anything different locally to actually start implementing that.

"We also have a few task forces for evidence review, so participating in that once-a-week sharing with a couple of committees locally to make sure, across the city and across the region, we're implementing the best care and the best policies for patients."

For Lynora Saxinger it was a task force, Alberta's Scientific Advisory Group, that required a lot of Covid research. "A lot of those hours I was spending looking at public health epi[demiological] reports and public literature and pre-prints and everything else. A lot of that time was trying to figure out answers to questions everyone was asking, so in some ways it was easy to pivot into saying yes to media requests because I didn't really have to prep. I was always marinating in this information, and I would relay what I could, so it was quite a pragmatic way to start."

But for all these doctors, it's about finding the time when you can. Lisa Barrett says, "You check up on things every hour, to be honest, and then you do your academic check once a day. Also, I'm not a sleeper—probably five hours pre-Covid times, probably about four hours now—so you have that hour before you go to bed when you just scan a whole lot of things, and you learn to get very good at knowing what is going to be important."

These are, I assume, skills that doctors hone in their training: what to pay attention to and how to retain it. And there's one other thing Barrett says that almost every person in this book has pointed out: "You can't keep up on every-thing, so the other piece is acknowledging what you don't know, the uncertainty of it." That candour, which I heard many times on and off the air, serves our audiences well.

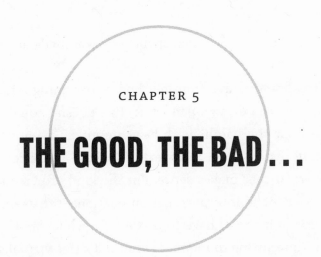

CHAPTER 5

THE GOOD, THE BAD . . .

IN 2019, MOST OF US HAD NEVER HEARD THE NAME LYNORA Saxinger. Now, lots of people across Canada know who she is, what she looks like, and have caught little glimpses of her personality, all through a small lens and microphone in her home office.

"It's actually been very very strange," she says. "If you pause to think how many people see that, it's paralyzingly terrifying. So in actual fact I'm just talking to a tiny little camera perched on top of my computer. On really busy days I'm running from one thing to another and it's, 'whoops,' put on some lipstick and a scarf and, boom. It was so busy I got acclimatized to it and I thought, 'All I can do is my best and move on.' I've become less stressed about it, but if I paused to think about it at all, it is kind of stressful because it's a lot of eyes.

"I'll actually try to not see myself. I'll watch the news but then I'll duck out for myself because it's so cringe inducing. I just can't. And if I watch, I think, 'I have to water that plant,' which I brought in because of the joke you made about my blank wall."

Broadcasting live from her house, becoming a trusted national voice during a pandemic, this doesn't come easily. But at least she's alone with her computer. "I am actually officially tested as an introvert, as a kind of extroverted introvert, if that makes sense. I'm the kind of person that, if I have a lot of interpersonal interactions, can seem very outgoing, but then I have to turtle for a while. So it's been kind of interesting to me that because it's this virtual space, it actually doesn't affect me as much as speaking to a group of people would."

It is through that camera lens that hundreds of thousands of people have looked inside her home, listened to her words and formed opinions about who she is and what she says.

"Does it feel like an invasion of privacy? Not at the time. I've actually had people say, 'I noticed you did the news from somewhere else in your house the other day,' and I think that's crazy. It's like this weird all-seeing eye you can manage not to think about too much, but you realize a lot of people watch it.

"I got recognized walking my dog the other day, and a patient I was seeing in clinic who actually had Lyme disease blushed when I came in to meet her. I don't know if I find that positive or massively strange, because I'm just an infectious diseases doctor.

"I do appreciate having people reach out and say the way I've said something or the way I've explained something is helpful for them. I do get that kind of feedback sometimes, and I do squirrel it away for down days. There are a lot of people who are consumers, they watch the flow. They don't always reach out, and when people reach out it's usually with a big positive or a big negative. But I think even with those extremes there have been more positives than negatives, and I think that's been helpful to me."

I ask what reaction she gets from her family. She says her parents "are just tickled to death. They just love it." It's also had an impact on her clinical practice, she jokes. "I have a lot of patients who listen to me more than they used to because I've been verified by CBC. One thing that I've noticed very very much is that my family will say, 'You look kind of tired' or 'You look very good.' They don't really comment on what I've talked about. It is nice. It's kind of cute. They probably have a better idea of what I do now than they ever did before, although it's all around one disease."

In Vancouver, Srinivas Murthy sometimes gets stopped at the grocery store by people who recognize him as "that doctor from TV," though, he notes, "I haven't got any autograph requests."

He also knows they're watching back home in Newfoundland. "My high school—Prince of Wales Collegiate—they all reached out and sent me an award," he says, laughing, reading from the email that described him as "Most Likely to Save the World from a Global Pandemic."

He says sometimes his family will text him while he's on the radio. Fortunately, he's resisted the impulse to throw in a word that would be a coded greeting, and, I was relieved to learn, he's withstood similar pressure from some of his friends. "They try to coach me into saying something stupid just to embarrass myself. I haven't done that yet. They'll give me sample words to say, like, 'Try to work the word "leapfrog" into your next thing, or "lilypad."' I try to work it in but never get to it."

I was surprised to hear Lisa Barrett doesn't get approached very much in Halifax. Surprised because her media appearances have made her very visible in the relatively small city. She says part of that may be because she is behind a mask all the time, but just as likely it's the respectful distance her fellow Maritimers would give any celebrity. "At the supermarket once I get to the checkout, or in the apartment building where I live, people will just pass by and say, 'Thank you for everything,' or something like that."

She says she was at a spa recently when one of the employees said a customer wanted to meet her but was too shy to come over. With a laugh she tells me, "I was, like, this is crazy. I'm just the doctor up the road."

And what about Isaac Bogoch? Public recognition is not something he mentions in our first two phone interviews, and when I ask him directly in a follow-up, he seems slightly uncomfortable with the subject. "I get recognized from time to time, at a grocery store or if I'm at a park with my kids. It happens. But, in all fairness, I stay pretty close to home. My kids did have a few questions when a stranger wanted to take a selfie with me while we were on a bike ride. It's . . . I mean." He pauses. "I'll chat with people. I'm obviously very appreciative. It's lovely that most people who do stop me say thank you, and I think that's very kind of them. It's not an annoyance whatsoever. I really do appreciate it."

Sumon Chakrabarti says, "People at my hospital recognize me. I'll get a patient who's seen me. They tend to be older." (Thanks for pointing out the TV news demographic, Sumon.) "It's been nice. I've not been embroiled in any kind of controversial battles, Twitter battles, any of that kind of stuff."

The doctors have done so many interviews in so many settings, and they haven't just offered up their expertise. They're often opening up their lives to the public. On the Sunday before Halloween, for example, Susy Hota was on *Cross Country Checkup*. We asked her to stay with us for ninety minutes and answer questions from callers about how to make trick-or-treating as Covid-safe as possible. Problem was, virtually no one had questions. Instead, they phoned in to tell great stories about how they were approaching this pandemic Halloween with care and creativity. Hota was patient and gracious, occasionally jumping in to tell people how great their ideas were and how she might try them with her own daughters. It was a good episode except for one thing. I worried that Hota would feel she had wasted her Sunday afternoon. Months later, I ask her how she felt that day. "I thought it was a really fun show," she says. "I remember it well, and I remember thinking, 'I really wish I could see that one house,'" referring to a caller in Toronto who described in detail an ambitious, colourful Halloween display.

She continues, "I think it's good in a way. I mean, sure, our time is precious, everybody's time is precious, and I agreed to do the show, I'm happy to do the show, and if there is a question or two that actually has to do with my area of expertise, I'm there to answer it. And the rest of the time, I think it's important for the public to see we're real people too. We aren't just the robots who are telling everybody to stay at home and wash their hands and wear masks for the rest of their lives. Sometimes there's a bit of a negative perception that the experts making the recommendations, they're so disconnected from what's actually happening in real life, and that's not the truth at all."

Allowing the people to see the "real" you can lead to some nice public interactions. During one of Lynora Saxinger's appearances in May 2021, a couple of callers made a point of thanking her for the advice she'd given during the pandemic. They spoke to her not as a generic expert, but almost as if she were a friend. Saxinger noticed that too. In an email she tells me:

> I have had similar experiences where people reach out in various ways and seem to feel like they know me, and generally there's an implicit gratitude for the connection. I think there are factors that contribute: maybe communication style, maybe being a woman, having a self-deprecating—wry sense of humour, being willing to reveal a bit of myself to connect (I've always done that as a doctor although not everyone does—it's a decision around professional veneer vs authenticity), not really being terribly interested in making myself sound intellectual in favour of trying to communicate accessibly.

I don't know how common that is but I'd assume
some of my colleagues, who are awesome, likely have
had similar experiences.

It's nice—I like people, and really those moments
help reassure that the time spent is worth it. I cer-
tainly try to weigh that greater than the less nice
"you'll be jailed with Fauci" nonsense (which would
be cool, actually), or getting copies of the Nuremberg
principles so I can defend myself in court for promot-
ing vaccination . . .

As those last comments reveal, not all contact with the public is smiles and virtual hugs. I ask Saxinger about the ugly reaction. "It usually peaks around discussion about lockdown. Some of [the extreme messages] can be super confusing. One of the first emails that made me go 'That's unpleasant' had 'commie Nazi,' then rude words for females that start with c, and I was just, like, 'wow.'" As she tells me the story, she jokes, "For one thing, I thought, 'You're very politically unaware. Those aren't usually the words that go together.'"

Like all the doctors, she says most of her feedback is positive, or at least neutral. "I get lots of emails that are try-ing to be helpful. For example, questions or advice about ivermectin [an anti-parasitic drug that was seen as a poten-tial Covid treatment], and if I have time to respond, I will. But some things can be disturbing. Overall, they're pretty rare. It's nothing compared to what people in public health get. But it's still nasty to think that people would actually reach out and think to share that. I do have a filter on my email now that pulls things out with certain keywords so it won't pop up while I'm on a Zoom call."

She says she sometimes checks what is in that filter because the university has asked her to see if there's anything coming in that could be a threat or otherwise makes her feel unsafe. When she spoke to me in late spring 2021, that hadn't happened.

Saxinger says sometimes she engages with the less nasty critics. "There are some people who kind of come out swinging. If you don't swing back, and leave some space to have a conversation, I've had a few times where people have been receptive to information. I don't always have the energy for that, but occasionally, if I'm feeling feisty. The key is to leave a space. For example, saying, 'I understand why people are worried about that. It's a very common worry. Here's why I don't think this is as big a concern as you think it is.'"

As a journalist, I sometimes go back and forth with viewers who send in angry criticisms, but I feel that what Saxinger is doing is different. I'm debating with them. She is a doctor who's used to dealing with difficult patients and is taking the time to try to help them. "Methodologically, you have to be in the right Zen headspace to engage. Otherwise you're best to ignore it. I went through a stage where I was trying to save the world because," she laughs, "that's how I manifest stress, apparently."

Srinivas Murthy sometimes replies to the public as well. "I've gotten thoughtful critical emails. People who will say,

'I've read the science and why haven't you said this?' I might respond politely or I might ignore it. I get a few a week, nothing more than that. They'll go in surges depending on how visible I am."

As for more negative emails, Murthy says, "I'll be frank and say I haven't got a ton of criticism of the things I've said. Whether that's because I'm even-keeled or I'm not inflaming the right people or I'm too quiet or something else, I don't know. But compared to friends of mine who do these things, I'll say that I have been limited in the amount of trolling I get online or in person."

Lisa Barrett says the feedback she has received on social media and in work and personal email has been overwhelmingly positive. The "negative bits"? "Less than 10 per cent. And people as often as not will have their own question added to the feedback, or they'll have an idea that they feel is very important on how we go forward, and that is never brought up in a negative way. I've gotten emails from all over Canada, from the US, from the UK, and people always want to share ideas. Thirty or forty per cent of the emails with messages have an acknowledgement that they feel they can share it with me. They feel comfortable sharing it. 'You seem like you're approachable' or something along those lines."

She says the criticisms that stick with her, interestingly, "are the people who seem reasonable because you think, 'Gosh, maybe I'm on the wrong track here.' I love hearing feedback on 'Maybe you can word this a little differently,'

'Make sure you mention this.' I love that kind of feedback. It's the minority, but I appreciate it."

As for the most common feedback? "I don't like it but I'll tell you anyway—it's people who say they find me calm. And I don't know if that's good or bad. But people seem to like a little bit of calm in their lives, and I think sometimes that's okay."

Why doesn't she like it?

"I find it boring. Who wants to be calm? One of the broadcasters, after we finished our segment, said, 'You have a velvet hammer. It was only afterwards I realized you just called someone out and no one really knew, as you smiled through it, that's what you were doing until they processed it a month later.'"

And then there are the rare but disturbing threatening emails. I want to stress that none of the doctors brought these up with me. But I did ask specific questions about this because I feel it's important to get a full picture of what they deal with. In Barrett's case, "I probably had about ten emails I've reported to local law enforcement, just in case something goes wrong, because it's completely out of the realm of rational." She pauses for a moment, then adds, "Which I actually think is pretty good, it's that infrequent."

Like all the doctors, she talks about the nasty emails quite matter-of-factly. I ask her if any left her shaken. "One email did. It was very, yeah, it was probably." She pauses to figure out how to describe it. "It was—the police thought it was more damaging than I did but, you know, personal threat and death and all that stuff and not in a gentle way."

Fatima Kakkar has also received a death threat during the pandemic, but it didn't have anything to do with her public profile. "It came straight from one of my patients' parents because I wouldn't write a letter of exemption. They wanted to have their child not to wear a mask in school. There's really no medical reason for that." So yes, it was a death threat, and yes, Kakkar says you do have to take that seriously. But she doesn't sound like she felt unsafe. "You know the patient, you know the family."

Beyond that incident, she says, "As far as social media, we take it with a grain of salt because we know we're going to be wrong on some fronts, and not let it cloud our day-to-day practice because there are so many opinions about Covid. There are such extreme opinions there is no way to appease everybody. I let it slide."

Alex Wong's assessment of public feedback? "Yes, there are weird people. There are people who like you and people who don't like you. I think I have the ability to objectively evaluate criticism from different people and from different forums. Then I'll decide if the criticism is something I need to respond to."

I ask if anything had crossed the line—in terms of race, for example. "I have not had anyone imply anything racist, overtly or not overtly." He did get some enraged reaction when he tweeted that Saskatchewan might want to follow BC's lead and not renew driver's licences for unpaid Covid fines. "I literally have people right now calling me a Nazi. Has it occurred to you that I'm not a white person? Am I even allowed to be a Nazi?"

Or as he tweeted:

> My email tonight:
> "All political, regulatory and medical actors
> involved in COVID-19 vaccination should
> familiarize themselves with the Nuremberg
> code and other legal provisions in order to
> protect themselves."
> I'm a Nazi? Have you seen me? C'mon, I'm a
> bald Asian midget, man.

But again, most of the feedback the doctors talk about has been encouraging. Zain Chagla says, "People tell me they appreciate my ability to communicate science. It was still science but it was more palatable and digestible to the general public, and making it much more relevant rather than being bombarded with high-level scientific language.

"I'm interested in what people think. Being a doc, you've had patients who disagree with you, patients who are extremely belligerent but you have to provide care for, and you get an extremely thick skin."

It didn't take long for the doctors to recognize which topics would bring in the most negative reaction. But Chagla says sometimes it can still come as a surprise. In April 2021 he was interviewed for an article in *Slate* on outdoor masking and thought, "'Oh, this is simple.' We don't do this much in Canada, we only do it in certain circumstances. In the US it's a massive thing, and places in Brooklyn, apparently, people get dirty stares on the streets if they don't wear their mask from the time they leave their front door until they return.

"So the author posted that article and people were infuriated by it. To me it seemed like a very reasonable article but, yeah, it was one of those things I got quoted on, and it was, 'Oh God, I didn't know this was this much a trigger point for people.' I think we live so reasonably here in Canada for our rules and restrictions."

I ask Chagla about the angry responses.

"Yeah, people quoting me and saying, 'This guy doesn't know what he's talking about,' and I'm like, huh, I didn't even think this was a thing, right? I thought we all understood the science of outdoors. Not necessarily that it was a mask mandate issue, but the ventilation is better and there's low risk . . . but clearly I was wrong.

"Whatever you say, there's going to be a side that doesn't agree with you, and because this pandemic has been so politicized, it's hard to always thread the line of what's science based and what's political or bias based. Everyone who reads those opinions goes to it with their own biases as opposed to taking it as objective or differing opinions."

I ask Chagla the same question I asked his colleagues: do the responses ever cross the line?

"There are certainly some Twitter trolls out there who will call us some very disgusting names or call us murderers. But there hasn't been direct racism. I don't think I've gotten a ton of direct racist stuff.

"I can say it bewilders me when all of us—ten-plus years trained, ten-plus years in clinical practice, constantly looking at the evolving evidence every day—that someone dismisses us, saying, 'You're completely wrong because I saw this YouTube video.' It's almost funny when you read through some of this. There is an argument for people getting critical thinking skills in high school and learning what is a legitimate source of information. I don't get mad about it, but it's funny how sure some people are of a particular issue in the pandemic. The best communicators are the most uncertain and the least able to make a complete assertion, because we all know there's some uncertainty in the evidence."

Chakrabarti also says most of what he hears is positive. "People that I know have been very good. To be honest with you, multiple times people have said, 'I trust what you tell us because I know if it's something bad, you'll tell us, but you're also putting it into context.' If I've ever had bad feedback, nasty feedback, it's just Twitter trolls, because I don't wade into politics. I'm not a really controversial guy."

I wonder if that "nasty feedback" ever gets racist. "Yeah. I get a lot of weird emails. They're more weird than anything. Of course, the garden variety 'Go back to where you came from' or 'You guys smell like curry.'"

Chakrabarti's perspective on those kinds of comments may surprise some people. "I don't mind saying to you that while this stuff sucks, I think it can be blown out of proportion. The people who are saying this are random. You know, those eggs on Twitter when you don't have a profile picture [an egg is a generic Twitter symbol that often denotes an anonymous account]. It's not like I'm going on TV and an anchor is saying something racist, or someone I know in person.

"I grew up in Sarnia in the '80s. I had friends who were curb stomped. I was bullied by Nazi skinheads. Racism, of course, exists, but calling what's happening to me now racism would be unfair to what actually happened before. [The ugly feedback now] has not had any influence on me."

Susy Hota has received "some bizarre, unusual emails. Eyebrow raising . . . but essentially harmless." She says one time she got a voicemail that was "very threatening sounding but didn't issue a threat to me, but I did report it because I was told I should do that."

She says she's had "a couple of emails, there was one recently that was fairly critical and . . ." she pauses, "frankly inappropriate how they characterized me, but, yeah, I don't know. I read those kinds of things and see angry, fearful, confused people. I think that just further motivates me to try and get the message out, and maybe work harder the next time I try to make a message around the vaccine, or whatever it may be, to be a little more mindful of how people react.

"You do the best you can around some of these topics. The information changes the next day and you can look like a bit of a dolt for saying something, but that was the truth of the matter as it stood at that time. And some people just have their entrenched beliefs about things, and it doesn't matter what I would say or what anyone else would say. They will always feel that way. So, I don't know. At times it can bother me. At other times I find it just rolls off my back and I realize it doesn't warrant the time to be worried about it."

Interestingly, the backlash that really bothers Hota is from "people you'd consider your colleagues." For example, when "there are implications that outbreaks have occurred in my hospital because of deficient practices or things that were done incorrectly. They're very careful to not name me specifically, but tagging me on things and making me very easily identifiable that if there's a criticism of what's happening in my hospital, it's directed towards me."

She says the way it has sometimes been expressed "is just not okay. We should have debates and encourage different opinions, but it should never get personal. And it should also never be undermining credibility, saying it in a way that questions your legitimacy. I have had some junior female colleagues with a shaky voice worried they were going to lose their jobs.

"When I do see people try to attack the reputation of my colleagues or other people who do the work that I do, mainly because they don't understand, I think that's incredibly unfair and that bothers me. So seeing the attacks on others who I know are trying to do the best they can with everyone's interests in mind, I think it bothers me more than some of these personal attacks from people who have their own beliefs."

Zain Chagla has had a similar experience. "There are people that want a particular message out there. Many of us try to be non-partisan and display the science, but there are people who want to take a line based on their ideology." And that, he says, has created divisions in the medical and science communities. "There's definitely been negative feedback from colleagues, and usually you can trace it back to bias or a personal argument, but generally I think most people have been pretty encouraging and feel that having balanced messaging is so important. There are obviously people who send messages to say, 'You're not saying things appropriately' or 'You're conveying the wrong message,' 'You're reckless,' that kind of thing. Of course you can have a different opinion. That's fine, that's debate. But you can also get a sense there's personal bias that drives that kind of feedback."

Hota agrees: "It's the worst when it comes from people you consider colleagues, peers or academics. That's actually hugely problematic and it's one of the reasons I don't engage on Twitter. The motivation behind [the criticism] is very concerning to me. It bothers me too because I'm a big believer in professionalism and respect and everything we're trying to promote—not just at my hospital but the University of Toronto and other academic institutions. This is a focus along with equity, inclusion, all of that. And yet we're in an era where we allow people who are fellow academics to behave that way, and it's really hard to call them on it and for there to be a consequence.

"In my case, this group has been less personal, not 'Susy Hota, you're an idiot, you don't know what you're doing.' However, what they've done is called me and my colleagues— those of us who do hospital infection prevention and control, a very small group of us—they have called into question our competency, our intentions in setting policies, accusing us of not protecting people enough, being slow, backwards, unresponsive, science-denier, which are the complete opposite of the truth. And so general terms like that, or connotations in their tweets or postings, you know, the public and other people who have no idea what we actually do—I mean, gosh, who knows what infection prevention and control is?—could easily take that and see very biased, cherry-picked information that seems to substantiate [the criticism], and draw conclusions that I think are very harmful, especially during a pandemic when we are in the middle of a lot of work that's happening and the response.

"It's not productive. It's very harmful because it's a very slanted argument, and what's hard about it is those of us who disagree and are in the middle of it and are being targeted in that sense, professionally, know that if we engage, it just gets worse. So we've been silent. And it's, like, 'You've not defended yourself in this court of public opinion,' but it's not the right thing to engage.

"In what I do in infection prevention and control, I rely on influencing people as the main mechanism of changing behaviour so we can have a safer environment. That's really what it is. It's soft science, and it's not your traditional medical sciences. You have to persuade people to wear their personal protective equipment properly, every time. How do you do that? Some of it has to be with behaviour change. How do you influence that? You have to have their trust. So your reputation, your credibility and the way that you explain things to people is so incredibly important. So when you have colleagues who are highly regarded, and have a lot of followers, implying that you are not a credible individual in what you do, and what you do in a professional sense is a piece of crap, and it's laughable—it basically has the potential of taking down the entire profession. You lose whatever ability you have to speak to the people you need to speak to. So it can be really dangerous in that respect."

Isaac Bogoch also spoke about the divisions among professionals—his comments are in the next chapter. As for feedback from the public, it probably won't surprise you to hear that the most high profile of the doctors receives many positive comments and some disturbing ones as well. "I get emails. Some of it is very lovely and nice. Some of it is pretty disparaging." He laughs. "Some days I'm a shill for [Canadian prime minister] Trudeau, other days I'm a shill for [Ontario premier] Doug Ford, but every day I'm a dirty Jew."

I wasn't prepared for how that sentence ends, but Bogoch doesn't seem too disturbed. "There's a lot of antisemitism but, really, I can block it and I can delete and I can move on with my life. It's annoying, but it truly doesn't impact my day-to-day life. I can't explain why." He laughs again. "Maybe it's growing up the middle child and getting abuse from all sides and playing hockey for a million years and the trash talking. I'm just used to it and, honestly, Ian, in a sick sick way, I get a sense of pleasure. You sort of stop and think, 'This is crazy . . .' and move along."

I ask if it ever bothered him. His answer? "Once." And then he reveals this unsettling story. "There were credible death threats. I was at home. This was early in the pandemic. I was on my phone and it was like it had crossed the boundary between online harassment to where there might be something more here. I remember thinking to myself, 'Okay, shit.' The two things that came to my mind were, number one, 'I've got to call the police,' and number two, 'How the hell am I going to walk downstairs, talk to my wife about this,' as my wife and kids were downstairs."

Despite the subject matter, Bogoch is describing this as if he were telling a story about a dramatic moment on a fishing trip. "I took a moment to collect my thoughts. I remember walking downstairs and saying, 'Uh, Linda, do you have a second?' I totally had the wrong delivery. I don't remember exactly what I said, but it was something like 'There's credible death threats, we probably should spend the night in a hotel and I'm going to call the police.'"

Bogoch is now laughing at how clumsily he felt he delivered the news. "My wife's jaw dropped. Right after that, I called the police. They were wonderful. They came over quickly. Of course, I had to have a conversation with the kids: 'There's police coming over and everything's okay and we'll be fine. Just let me chat with the police privately please.'

"The police took it very seriously. They had a police car parked outside our house for a couple of days. They looked at security camera footage from a lot of people in our neighbourhood, and they had extra cruisers. It was noticeable in our area for a while, and then it died down."

As comfortably as he tells the story, he also makes it clear: "When it starts to impact your family, obviously that's a major line to cross and that really upset me."

I ask if he knows what was behind the threat. "It's hard to know the motive. There was some antisemitic rhetoric. I don't know if that was the prime motivation, but it was certainly a component. 'We know where you live,' and there's some credible information that they do know where you are. The police said they were worried about it and they would take it seriously and they did. They were terrific."

To be clear, Bogoch only tells me this story when I specifically ask about negative feedback and whether it ever made him uncomfortable. And despite this one troubling threat, he tells me he did not consider this a significant problem for him. "There are some of my colleagues who are getting the same degree of harassment, be it through their gender or their religion or their political opinions—we all are. And we hear that women bear the brunt of this more significantly than men. Racialized professionals bear the brunt of this as well. I would never want to underplay how significantly this affects other people. And I know other people have been so disturbed they've taken a step back at times, and I completely respect that. But for me, personally, I'm not trying to present a brave face. Minus the death threat, I just don't give a shit. I truly don't care. And I can move on with my life.

"Some people copy and paste it and put the threat online. I could do this lots of times a day, but I don't because for me, at least, that's not the issue. The issue is, let's deal with this damn pandemic and move on with our lives. It really isn't about me."

CHAPTER 6

SENDING A MESSAGE

IT WAS SUNDAY, JANUARY 24, 2021. THE *NATIONAL TALK* team was brainstorming what topics to focus on for another edition of "Doc Talk," our informal name for the segments where one or two doctors would answer questions—sometimes from viewers, sometimes from us. I had an idea and did a quick search of our archives to confirm my hunch: it had been fifty-two weeks since my first Covid interviews with Isaac Bogoch. I suggested to our team that we ask him and Lynora Saxinger, the second doctor I'd interviewed, to reflect on events of the past year. Not just what we'd learned about the science of Covid, but also their own experiences, what it was like to step into the national spotlight during a pandemic. You'll recognize this as a topic I'm interested in: it became the theme of this book. You never know how these pitches will go—lots of people bring their own suggestions. But, fortunately, my colleagues liked the idea.

So, how was that first year? Here's part of what Saxinger said on the show: "I guess I now realize how many people watch the news because I realize people feel they know me, and I've had a lot of nice interchanges with people who say thank you for the information and thank you for making it easier to understand."

Bogoch concurred. "I think I've had a similar experience as Dr. Saxinger. The occasional nod [in public], the occasional smile, the occasional very kind comment. It's wonderful to see."

But I was a little worried. After the taping I asked them, as I usually do, if they were happy with how it went. Saxinger said it was okay, but, based on her tone, I wasn't sure. Screening the interview, I thought it went well. But later that night I looked at Saxinger's Twitter feed and discovered—or at least I think I discovered—why she seemed pensive after the taping. She tweeted there was a lot more she wanted to say:

> As usual I had lots of thoughts AFTER . . .
> (sigh) but hey, we just had a few minutes. A
> few extra ponderings about 2020:

Tweets are short—there's a limit of 280 characters. But you can thread together a series of tweets, and that's what Saxinger did, covering a range of topics she didn't get to on *The National* earlier in the evening, from the disruption and stress of the pandemic to her motivation for engaging with media:

> I could see an influx of conspiracy theories,
> and misweighting of the significance of new

> research, and thought—if I don't pitch in
> where I see possible problems, I couldn't
> forgive myself

And she included some very personal reflections.

> So, how was the year? I gained weight
> from sitting at my computer reading and
> synthesizing until all hours and stress eating.
> My family deserves medals. My long term
> patients found me distracted but (maybe
> because I am on the news) . . . seemed to
> listen to my advice more (?!). I had a lot of
> hair fall out in about April-June (telogen
> effluvium), and learned not to read the
> comment section.

Since then I've watched her Twitter feed closely, enjoying the unique mixture of medical data, personal reflections, cat news ("*18 pounds of badly timed affection comes to lie on the keyboard*") and humour. Unlike those many media interviews that brought the infectious disease docs to public attention, social media has given them their own direct channel to connect with tens of thousands of people.

If you follow Saxinger, you've come to expect life observations like this:

> Dear world, I legit do not SUGGEST using
> a mask walking alone ordinarily, but I

am between buildings and it's snowing
a bit and really windy and I wish it also
covered my ears.

Or a comment, illustrated by a photo of a US politician
with a mug of beer:

Whether you "observe" St. Patrick's Day
or not, a moment of silence for this terrible,
terrible looking pint hoisted by Paul Ryan a
few years back.

Was it poured hours before? Was it flat
root beer? I genuinely like Guinness and
this is sad.

Even typos lead to quips:

One day I'll stop tweeting from my phone,
and will also proofread.
Today is not that day.

Twitter allows people to toggle between lighthearted
and very serious, and that's what Saxinger does. From post-
ing data to try to counter misinformation:

Since the beginning of April:
97% of ICU cases were not immunized

> 98% of hospitalized cases were not
> immunized.
> (from 2 weeks post dose 1)

Or, on occasion, sending out a thread of tweets with a forceful message:

> I'm angry at the FLOOD of toxic
> misinformation that is being spread about
> COVID vaccines because it's actually
> murderous . . . people in their 70s with
> immune compromise in a city with >
> 200/100000 COVID cases weekly are
> AFRAID OF LIFE SAVING VACCINES . . .
> example absolute BS:

> I'm flabbergasted about the froth reach
> and number of Youtube videos, elder email
> chains, Facebook ridiculousness—like where
> did this all come from, why do they want
> people afraid and at risk? The vaccines are
> REALLY GOOD and better tested than most
> medicines people take . . .

> (FWIW froth was an autocorrect but not
> really bad enough to redo because . . . it
> is froth. Like rabid animal saliva froth or
> churned up soapy nonsense froth.)

> I'm becoming a conspiracy theorist now too.
> Why would such damaging misinformation
> be churned out like this? It absolutely
> undermines whole nations. It's vile. Please
> don't sit back. Stomp it out. Like you'd
> stomp flames in dry grass or cockroaches if
> you're not against that.

> Because this is a big deal. People are afraid
> of some of the best science I've seen, from
> scientists and technologists who were under
> the same pandemic threat as all of us. This
> is ridiculous. The vaccines are so damn
> good. We need to take them to protect
> selves—others.

By mid-June 2021, Saxinger had 22,000 Twitter followers. That's a pretty significant audience of people who have made the choice to receive her updates. You get some sense of the impact of that last tweet by the number of people who retweeted it to their followers (231) and publicly "liked" it (760), beyond all or most of the 20,000 who would have seen it.

That thread she sent out after our interview in January got a lot of supportive comments.

> I've enjoyed your calm demeanour on CBC.
> You never seem angry at the idiots who seem
> to roam the streets!

> Thank you for your explanations and insights.
> We depend on trusted professionals like
> yourself. You bring us honesty, clarity,
> reason, candour and comfort during a most
> challenging time. Stay well!

Saxinger says, "I was a Twitter neophyte before this thing started. I only had five hundred followers at most in the fall when I started toe-dipping into more professional-type Twitter." Pre-pandemic, Twitter was essentially a professional gathering place for Saxinger: "Some people had embraced Twitter as a vehicle for scientific linking and communication. I found some scientific information that was useful and then I transitioned more to public communication."

She admits that as public interest in the pandemic, and her following on Twitter, grew, "I went through a phase where I probably paid more attention to Twitter than I should have. I think there is a consuming-ness to the fast-paced information flow and the little clicks and all this kind of stuff that can become too engrossing. So I went through a phase of getting too intertwined in this Twitter-sphere and then backed away from it." As I hear her over the phone, I can imagine her speaking with a wry smile. "I think I'm over the acute phase."

A Sunday night in March 2021 was one of those times when it became, for a while, too much:

> Not sure what's up—some kind of
> zeitgeistian badness, an existential plague?

> But my Twitter feed is fully toxic and I will
> be spending less time for a bit. I'll come
> for the science but leave for the politics or
> yelliness. (Be nice, make good choices, walk
> outside a bit).

But that led to dozens of supportive comments, and soon she was back to it.

Her social media strategy? "Sometimes I'll do a tweet thread when I'm getting questions. For example, second-dose delay. I'll try to do one answer. It [social media] is in a way a little more reactive, and my Twitter use goes up and down. Sometimes I'll react to misinformation that I perceive is starting to get more capture. It's not about trying to promote an idea, per se.

"The other thing I do on Twitter lately is I let down my guard, and I'm just more me more often. It's just too exhausting keeping track of having more than one persona, so I'm just whatever this is, the way it is."

Saxinger has built a community of people who, based on their comments, like her and what she says. Besides the Covid information, they also get unfiltered glimpses of the personality behind the professional. Saxinger says, "I do find putting up quirky things or cat pictures, it really makes people feel like they know you, so you get a lot more positive personal interaction."

I ask her, "Did you ever think a year ago you'd post cat pictures?"

Her answer, leaving us both laughing: "No . . . it just tells me my psyche is broken down."

Isaac Bogoch is also relatively new to Twitter, and he's taken a very different approach. If Saxinger has curated a version of her complex self on social media, Bogoch has created a powerful news channel. The slogan could be "Almost all Covid, almost all the time."

He didn't have an account two years ago and says colleagues told him he should join. Since the pandemic, his number of followers has grown at an astonishing pace. Bogoch has taken a very disciplined approach to the social media platform. "Twitter is just an extension of what I've been trying to do in mainstream media, which is, number one, keep it business. My Twitter is very much science medicine, infectious diseases and public health. There's an occasional hockey and an occasional chicken wing [yes, he very occasionally tweets about the snack food]—but mostly work related. I don't veer off into arguing with anonymous individuals or robots. I don't opine on issues I really feel strongly about but I'm not a professional in. I read the newspaper. I have strong opinions. I just don't use Twitter for that platform.

"I try to be as honest and transparent as possible and keep politics out of it as well. I'm not saying this is the right way to do it. There are lots of right ways to do it, but when you look at some people's media, social media, they have a medical and scientific opinion, but they also blend that in with politics as well, and I try to stay as apolitical as possible.

Sometimes an unpopular politician may have a good idea, and it's okay to say 'That's a good idea.' Sometimes a popular politician may have a terrible idea. It's okay to say, in a constructive and fair manner, to discuss that. I think that approach has helped. There are a lot of people in Canada. I think if you only speak to people in your ideological silo, you're only going to be speaking to a minority of the population, and we have to reach everyone with this."

His tweets clearly reach a lot of people. Updates like this one, from late May 2021, prompted more than 6,000 people to press the "like" button. That means they read it and chose to publicly show they agreed with it.

> 183,399 #COVID19 vaccines were administered in Ontario, as of 8pm today. You read that right . . . >183K, the most vaccines administered in the province in a single day. By far. Happy Victoria Day long weekend everyone.

Many of his tweets draw lots of comments, almost all of them strongly supportive or friendly.

> Dr. Bogoch, As we begin a long weekend, I want to thank you for all of your efforts on our collective behalf!! You and all of your healthcare workers deserve Gold medals for everything you've done for us!!! Please take time this weekend to kickback!!!!

Or, more succinctly,

> Have a great weekend Isaac you have
> earned it

As Bogoch says, when he assesses government policy it's from an infectious disease perspective, as opposed to a political perspective. Deep in the third wave, when the Saskatchewan government released a chart of its reopening plan, Bogoch retweeted the graphic and wrote:

> It is really helpful to see what the #COVID19 "off ramp" looks like. Saskatchewan's reopening plans are very clear, outlining estimated timelines, setting achievable & meaningful vaccine targets, with clear guidance.

Perhaps my CBC Vancouver colleague Justin McElroy, whose Covid charts have become famous here in British Columbia, could create a snazzy graph plotting Bogoch's skyrocketing Twitter impact. Early in the pandemic I seem to remember he was somewhere in the 40,000s. Every few weeks, like the totals during a telethon, his number of followers rose sharply. By June 2021 it was well over 120,000.

What that means is every tweet—well, maybe not the ones about chicken wings—but most of his tweets have an impact on the topic of his choosing. When he's on a news program, he defers to the interviewer. Not once has he suggested to me what to discuss. But in his Twitter community—which has as many people as a small Canadian city—he's in charge. (I've been trying to come up with a Sheriff Bogoch joke, but I don't want to detract from the serious journalistic analysis going on here.)

By almost any measure, when it comes to Covid in Canada, he would be considered a social media phenomenon. So his view of the platform might surprise you. "I'm very leery of Twitter. To put it on a scale of net benefit and net harm, I think it would tilt to the net harm side of the scale. There's just so much misinformation, there's a lot of amplification of pseudoscience, there's a lot of amplification of very polarizing beliefs that might slightly align with reality but don't entirely align with reality, and it's just a mess."

Having said that, he clearly spends time on the social media site. Sometimes at night in the Pacific time zone, I'll see him tweet, surprised he's up past midnight, eastern time. Still, you can see the limits he sets for himself. He follows fewer than a thousand accounts, limiting it to "infectious diseases, medicine, hockey—and Canadian Paintings—I love Canadian Paintings [@CanadaPaintings]. It is the best thing on Twitter." (He often will add one of the paintings featured on that account to his Ontario vaccination updates.)

Given his criticism of Twitter, I ask if his presence was a strategy to balance out the pseudoscience. "Oh yeah," he says. Drawing out the words again, for emphasis. "Oh. Yeah." As you read this section, imagine his tone on TV. Not angry. Just conversational. "Some of my colleagues are overtly wrong or choosing wilfully to ignore science or choosing wilfully to inflame a situation, and it's disgusting. This pandemic will come to an end, and there are people who will not be welcomed back. This is coming from otherwise smart people. A lot of people have lost their heads."

And so what is Bogoch's Twitter strategy? "If I see something I like, I'll retweet it. Most of the time I'll see something not on Twitter and I'll post it. An interesting study, updated medical advice. Or if I hear some very polarizing comments that are just inaccurate, I'll try to give some perspective to it. Then I'll scroll for a minute or two, and then I'll get annoyed or disgusted and I'll log out and move on with my day."

When we spoke, it was still relatively early in Ontario's vaccine rollout and a then current example came to mind: the criticism, reflected in some media coverage, that vaccines were languishing in freezers. "Nothing drives me more crazy than [criticizing] 'vaccines in freezers' because multiple things can be true. Can the province more rapidly vaccinate? Absolutely. Should the provinces have a better means to mobilize vaccines quickly into arms from when they get delivered? Sure, totally. But the second a vaccine is delivered, to take a snapshot right then and say there's 800,000 vaccines in freezers right after they're delivered is disingenuous, it's not a fair criticism and it doesn't really account for the complexities of . . ." He pauses for a second. "The vaccines get delivered, then they get mobilized around the province and then they have to go into arms. Both things can be true, but at least be honest and fair with your criticism. So things like that bother me, and that's just one of about 8 trillion examples where you're taking a 3 out of 10 problem and creating an 11 out of 10 problem." (For the record, comic hyperbole is a device he saves for book interviews, not interviews on *The National*.)

And on the more serious topic of negative Twitter reaction, he offers advice I wish I could follow: "I know that anyone who's public gets their fair share of abuse, and it will come through comments on Twitter—which I see from time to time and then I smile and ignore them. The beautiful thing about Twitter is all you have to do is turn it off and the problem goes away. It's as simple as that. It just doesn't bother me. People say terrible things and I just don't care. I can turn it off and move on with my life and that's the end of that."

By contrast, Bogoch's University Health Network colleague Susy Hota has stepped away from Twitter altogether. "I honestly cannot find the time or energy to do it because it's such a volatile environment." She laughs as she continues. "You can very easily offend someone or say something that can be taken and used against you, and I know that although I get lots of positive feedback and support from people, there are also people out there who are just waiting to jump at anything I say. And so it's just not worth that, to be honest. It's tough enough for all of us to get through this pandemic."

Srinivas Murthy is still on Twitter, but barely. He often goes days between tweets, and as I scroll through his posts, I see the topics are often global health and equitable access to vaccines. "I'm a low-volume engager," he tells me. "I don't do a lot of tweeting, and I'll respond to things either when, a., I'm passionate about them or, b., I want to publicize but not to engage in conversation that requires nuance." In his carefully understated way, Murthy adds, "I think that is not the space Twitter excels at. It's great to keep up to date with what's happening in Canada, the most recent numbers, follow a few source individuals, but to actually have a conversation about any specific approach, it's not for that."

On the other coast, Lisa Barrett is a fairly high-volume tweeter. When I ask her about feedback, she tells me, "I would say 80 per cent positive." Comments like this:

> You the Woman, Doctor Barrett!

> A voice of calm and reason.

> Your candid, honest and well informed
> tweets and interviews are my "go to" for
> balanced information. Have you ever
> thought of doing a podcast??

If you scroll through her tweets, you'll see her give the occasional piece of advice, like this one, to her fellow Nova Scotians, as the third wave surged:

> This virus is quick and quiet, and we will lose
> control fast. Bubbles that maximize what we
> are allowed to do are just a bit much for the
> next couple of weeks. Choose to stay home,
> NS. And not just in some areas. Viruses don't
> know about our political map marks.

She even sent a pointed message to her provincial government while that third wave was still underway:

> My idea of light at the end of the tunnel
> does NOT involve opening too soon. I hope
> Nova Scotia sticks to our numbers based,
> quantitative, cautious plan to re-opening
> that gets us back to a goal of no COVID
> community spread before opening. @nsgov

But most of her tweets, at least in the spring of 2021, were on widespread Covid testing:

> Get tested if it's available, people. Testing
> capacity without noses to swab because
> people feel they aren't the "risky person" is
> inaccurate (unless you live alone and never
> leave your house), dangerous, and harmful
> to KEEPING COVID cases low.

Barrett tells me, "I am very much an advocate of testing because I think we have a duty to keep our vaccines as effective as we can, and testing is important for that," but she says she didn't set out to make Twitter a platform for that advocacy. Instead, she wanted to complement the more traditional media approach of the health officials and "ended up co-opting my Twitter."

If anything has co-opted Sumon Chakrabarti's Twitter, it's tennis. The banner picture across the top shows one of the sport's legends, Rafael Nadal. Chakrabarti's timeline is heavy on Covid information, with a sprinkling of gifs and more tennis updates than absolutely necessary.

Like Saxinger, his personality is reflected in some of the more whimsical posts ("*Is there anything more wasteful than poppy seeds on a bagel*"), but he also uses the platform to bring attention to the Covid messages he finds important. For example, this tweet in April 2021:

> Outdoor transmission remains exceptionally rare and I am skeptical it occurs even in some crowded circumstances.

The topic of outdoor transmission came up a lot in my interviews for this book. In part that's because there was a lot of debate about it in the spring of 2021, when I spoke to the doctors. But it also provides a good illustration of what motivated them to engage with the public, especially on platforms like Twitter, where they can decide what to talk about.

Chakrabarti's take is that "there has been a lot of abstinence-based messaging. It was very frustrating for me. Yes, we had been in a really really bad situation, but people wanted to believe we should be in a bubble."

He remembers his reaction to seeing someone else's tweet "about the story of a person who was outside and got Covid and ended up in the ICU. That type of thing bothers me because it's an emotional anecdote that really really scares people, but it's not really representative of what's happening outdoors. Of course bad things happen. But, come on, guys, what the public is concluding is that it's unsafe to be outdoors, that if I go outdoors I'm going to end up on a ventilator. That particular comment was not productive."

As Chakrabarti explains: "There are two concepts I've noticed very very clearly throughout the entire pandemic. The first one is the idea of risk tolerance. People have moved towards zero risk, which is not realistic. I get it. If you're sitting close together outdoors, yeah, transmission could happen, but it's the visibility bias. If you break up a group and drive them indoors, the total number of cases that could happen from that is much higher than the people hanging out in a park.

"The second thing I've noticed is, and I don't quite know the word for it, but it's almost like people feel because you're in a pandemic, you can't do anything leisurely. Anything that has the appearance of leisure, whether it's skating outdoors, sitting outdoors in a park, people rain down anger on you. [But then] you think about last year, the Black Lives Matter protests. It's almost as if there was a disconnect in people's minds because Black Lives Matter was a cause we wanted to support. All of a sudden, that debate about infectious diseases and transmission went out the window. To be fair, there was no spike of transmission leading to hospitalizations from that. My point is, people were using their morals to interpret the situation rather than their objectivity."

And so he sent tweets like those below. As you read his tweets—or any doctor's tweets for that matter—keep in mind the two or three lines sum up a more complex analysis.

· Mother's Day weekend is coming up. We all
know the public health recommendations,
but I already see the shame-based,
abstinence-based messaging starting. In the
spirit of risk mitigation: if you do see your
mom this weekend and she's in a different
household . . . 1/

. . . keep the risk as low as possible by
staying outdoors (preferably the entire
time) and distanced. Keep the group small.
Also . . . flowers . . . lots of flowers :) Happy
Mother's day!

I ask him if he thinks his tweets on the topic had an impact.

"To be honest with you, it's hard to know. I got a lot of criticism for that tweet, mainly from people who are saying that I was discounting airborne transmission. The problem is on Twitter, you don't know the quiet majority who is listening to you. I did get a lot of personal messages asking me specific questions that show that they were informed by my tweet. I also got questions in the media about it, so I was able to amplify my message that way. Overall, I unfortunately think that Twitter is a bit of a necessary evil. I do it to keep up to date with new things that are happening, but I don't find it particularly useful for discussion."

Fatima Kakkar's Twitter experience reflects that of some of the other ID docs, beginning before the pandemic when she was using the platform to connect with other doctors and scientists. "Unlike other social media feeds, where it's personal, there's an academic Twitter and a medical Twitter and an ID Twitter to bring together these ID docs from around the world, and these are people that I've met at conferences. We review medical articles together, and someone puts up pre-publication prints of their article.

"There were many situations where I was ahead of the mainstream scientific reviews because so much was being published on Twitter, so for me, originally, it was more of a resource, staying in touch with my other ID colleagues around the world."

But, as it has for her colleagues, "more recently it's become more of a platform. The more you use it the more you realize you can say things that will have an impact."

She retweets articles of note and some snapshots of what she's seeing with patients:

> Thinking goggles, masks and PPE scare kids
> in clinic?
> Nope.
> 3 year-old leans in to give me a big old hug
> as I listen to his heart.
> I get 4 babies to smile from behind my mask.
> 4 year-old even laughs at my jokes.
> Kids adapt. This is #pediatrics in the time of
> #COVID19

Kakkar says, "It's been a learning process for me. I used to use it as a resource, but now I use it as a tool. But it's a little bit intimidating. It worries me that if I say something and someone takes my advice, will I be liable? But it's been terrific to be able to connect with all of these different groups. In the hospital I've been the one pushing my colleagues to get on Twitter. Our usual means of communication are press releases, web diaries and our journal publications, and they take so long that it's just not helpful in this pandemic. Twitter has been very positive. Yes, there's the occasional bad feedback, but I haven't had what a lot of people have had in terms of negative feedback."

Alex Wong says his first appearance on *The National*— which, coincidentally, was alongside Kakkar—was a turning point in his Twitter life. His profile states he was an early adopter, joining way back in 2010. But he says he didn't really become active on the social media platform until early 2021.

Even as his national profile grew, Wong focused his Twitter message on his home province. His strategy "kind of grew organically, and it became a way to advocate without being too political, and trying to provide a realistic and accurate perspective on what was really going on without people perceiving I was being influenced either by the health authority or by the government. For the most part, I hope it's been helpful."

He says that "with the third wave happening in Saskatchewan, and we had one of the highest proportions of variants in the country, that also became a bit of a rallying cry to fill a void. I didn't know who in the province was being relied on to provide clear evidence, clear facts." Wong describes his approach as "being humble enough to be able to say there are things we don't understand right now," and he points out that "taking things that are really complicated and trying to make them simple is not simple. If you say one thing that is not quite correct, or even correct but can be interpreted in different ways, that can lead to all kinds of angst."

Scroll through his tweets and you'll find a range of information. For example, when vaccine-induced immune thrombotic thrombocytopenia (VITT, rare blood clots associated with the AstraZeneca vaccine) was becoming a major news story, he posted:

> Apparently SK has its first case of VITT associated with AZ vaccine. NOT unexpected, NOT reason for alarm.

> Again, to provide reassurance, everyone who received 1st dose AZ: you ABSOLUTELY 100% made the right decision to get your 1st dose. More information coming.

During the third wave, Wong used Twitter to encourage people to reduce their risks:

> test positivity % in #SK continues to be stubbornly high. Positivity % in #YXE

continue to rise. So *definitely* not out of
woods yet. Critical for all of us to:
- vaccinate!
- tightest bubbles
- test & isolate
- be ++ safe
Love, Alex

Occasionally he tweeted some pointed criticism of political leaders:

Couldn't listen to presser b/c of work,
but consistent theme of shifting blame to
individual #SK citizens (get vaccinated!
stay at home! don't be stupid!) deliberately
shifts attention from those most directly
responsible: our elected leaders in
government. #COVID19SK

Wong says he doesn't use Twitter just to get his message out but also to learn from trusted sources. "Now that I'm following many of my colleagues, it's been easier to be comfortable and confident in my interpretation of the big picture because I can engage with my colleagues who are bright and see the micro-picture and the big picture. I know if I'm on the same page they are. So, for example, AstraZeneca, the timing of the second dose. There's a relatively clear answer to this: there's data uncertainty, and you have to explain risk/

benefit to the public. That's what it comes down to, so it's actually been a little easier for me now."

The more time he spends on social media, the more Wong says he's adjusting his approach to public communication. "I've been learning as we go about how all this works and how to engage people. I'm doing Q & A sessions now for two hundred or three hundred classes of Grade 8s. But I've also learned the need to repeat certain messages over and over. There are times where I'd do one interview and then another, and they'd ask the same questions again. It does get tiring, intellectually, to answer the same questions over and over again, but it's become very clear to me that you need to engage different media platforms, different people, because everyone has different preferences on how they get their information."

On Twitter, feedback can be instant and, as Wong says candidly, that can be both a good and bad thing. "For the most part it has been positive, and that makes me feel good. Positive reinforcement makes us all feel good, right? When I started engaging on Twitter in March [2021] I could tell how it was becoming addictive, it was almost like an endorphin rush. I was checking all the time, 'Oh my God, I've got this many followers, all these people saying nice things about me.' I quickly understood how this could be this never-ending rabbit hole where you dive down, so after a couple of days of that I thought, 'This is not sustainable. I clearly need to compartmentalize this aspect of my life.' At least I had enough awareness to do that."

And he is aware that getting on the many other social media platforms isn't practical. "I wish I had had time to engage on different social media platforms, like Instagram or Facebook or even, God forbid, TikTok. People have explained very clearly to me the different demographics and dynamics of how people communicate on these platforms. I just haven't had time."

So that's a hard no to the newest of social media, TikTok, but, like a lot of infectious disease doctors, he has on occasion turned to the oldest of the traditional media and written an op-ed for the newspaper.

The op-ed is a guest commentary, appearing on the page opposite the editorials written by the newspaper. It was, in the old days, a highly visible platform that would generate a lot of debate and discussion.

These days, of course, fewer people get a morning paper delivered to their home. But whether it's in print or online, the op-ed can still be influential, noted by journalists and shared by readers.

Like Twitter, it allows the infectious disease docs to send out their own message, as opposed to answering a journalist's questions and seeing their comment reduced to a short clip or quote in a news piece. But unlike Twitter, rather than being limited to 280 characters, you often have 600 to 800 words to make your point.

Wong reached out to the *Regina Leader-Post* to write a piece on the first anniversary of the pandemic. However, his focus wasn't on looking back. As the title makes clear, he was very much looking at the present situation: "Province Must Come Together to Fight Off a Potential Third Wave."

Wong tells me, "Once this third wave thing happened, when we learned our variant proportion in Saskatchewan was so high, like higher than pretty well everywhere else in the country outside of maybe northern Ontario, that was a real shock to us, and it was a leading indicator we were going to get smashed pretty badly, which we did. And it was also a leading indicator of what was going to happen in the rest of the country as well."

His op-ed was a careful combination of raising the alarm while still sounding optimistic, which is captured in the closing.

> I grew up in Ontario, did my post-graduate training in Alberta and began working full time in Regina in 2011. Much of what drew me to this province was the collective spirit of Saskatchewanians, the desire to do good by our provincial motto, Multis e gentibus vires—From Many Peoples Strength. We need to channel that collective spirit in this moment as we face our greatest threat. Please, follow the public health guidance, keep your personal and family bubbles extremely tight, isolate and test when symptomatic. And get vaccinated when it is your turn.

I was surprised to learn how quickly he was able to write the piece. Wong says, "Since at the time my brain was all COVID-19, all the time, the initial drafts probably took me less than an hour to bang out. Not long at all." His target wasn't just the public but also decision makers in Saskatchewan. In his usual self-deprecating style, Wong says, "Of course, I'm realistic in believing that none of it made a difference, but it's always hard to know how things exactly work in government, and I've also at times throughout the pandemic recognized that sometimes people were paying attention when I didn't think they were paying attention." He says the reaction was "generally positive, but with all things COVID-19, it faded quickly" as the ICU started filling up during the third wave.

A few weeks earlier, Saxinger had been invited by the *Calgary Herald* to write her own op-ed to mark the first anniversary of the pandemic. Her commentary is titled "After a Year of Widespread Loss and Now Hope, It's Time to Heal and Rebuild." She says she enjoyed the opportunity to be in control of the content and have more room to make her point. "One thing about being reactive and trying to answer questions is that you're not in your own space, you're actually in someone else's space, and it's a reactive space and that's fine. But being able to sit down and think about what my messaging is, and then compact it into the right number of words, I found it was a nice opportunity. I think the creation of something like that is very different from what I've been doing all along, and it felt a little bit cathartic, honestly."

Here's an excerpt of her reflections on the pandemic's impact on the public discourse:

Divisions that were under the surface are laid
bare, and so are the networks that pull groups both

farther into themselves and apart from each other. And these divisions have to heal too, although this certainly won't happen on Facebook, Twitter or in newspaper comment sections. We seem to have developed tribes, who consider each other completely deluded and wrong, and who may even hold each other largely responsible for the suffering the pandemic has brought. How will we get our sense of community back?

It is a powerful piece that doesn't pull punches. But as you'd expect from her, and as the title suggests, it ends with a sense of hope:

I am really looking forward to a few months from now, when we will be able to meet—with open minds and patient hearts—in real life, rather than in virtual silos and conflicts. In the fresh light of day, we will see again that we are all just people, doing our best through a bad time. And we will start to heal.

Boosted by the profile of major Canadian newspapers, and remaining forever just a Google search away, these op-eds can get a lot of scrutiny for a long time. Zain Chagla, who has co-written about one a month, says that can be daunting. "There's always that nervousness. Is there something we missed? That's why I don't write by myself. It's always good to get your biases checked. But there's always that feeling in the pit of your stomach. Will something come out in two months that completely refutes what I say, and I'll have this legacy in the public. But we try to be evidence based, at least the state of evidence at the time."

He says people have generally appreciated his pieces. "We're not writing a state of the union. It's an issue one of us has identified as a big problem that we really do want to change the narrative on, or help lead to a more nuanced discussion around the narrative. This is not us trying to be political commentators. We're trying to create an article with solutions and discussion points rather than blame and shame."

His first op-ed came a few months into the pandemic, in July 2020. It was co-written with Bogoch and Chakrabarti for the *National Post*. The title: "We're Infectious Disease Experts, and 'Eliminating' COVID Won't Happen Any Time Soon."

Chagla says the three of them had a rare moment where they not only had time to meet, but could also meet in person. You may remember, as we headed into the summer of 2020 and case counts fell, there was a sense of hope among some people that Canada might be able to stamp out Covid. Perhaps a strict lockdown for a few weeks could lead to life returning to normal. Chagla says he, Bogoch and Chakrabarti "had a drink together on a patio and just talked about what was going on. And I think one of the things that came out of that conversation was that people didn't have a concept this was a virus that was going to be incredibly difficult to contain. And based on the history of other infectious diseases, this was not something that was going to be eliminated off the earth.

"I think all three of us felt that message was being lost in everything, with flattening the curve, the initial 'do everything to get everything under control.' Not to say we wanted to ease restrictions and everyone be free again, but at the same time we wanted to really make people think about what the future was with this virus, more than just case counts and that kind of thing.

"I think that was one of the big messages, we really wanted to push the people to get a better sense of what the future looks like."

The op-ed ends with this statement:

> As infectious diseases physicians, we feel it is warranted to be honest with the population and caution against using the term "elimination" or "eradication" in the context of this disease and alleviate some of the anxiety and sense of failure with case counts ongoing in the community. We need to focus on using the correct language of containment, reduction and risk mitigation as part of the discussion moving forward, rather than elimination or eradication.

Op-eds generate streams of feedback, including online comments at the bottom of the article, people reacting on social media, and often discussions on news programs and podcasts. I ask Chagla about the reaction to the piece. "Some people took that message to heart and said it resonated with them because no one was talking about that." But, of course, there were negative comments. "Some people were really angered by it, and they made it seem that by putting that message out there we were somehow enabling a plan to live with the virus that didn't involve severe elimination. They felt that somehow that aspirational goal of elimination [of Covid] was being put aside because we were being very practical about this."

But the negative reaction didn't deter them. All three kept writing. Shortly before I interviewed them in 2021, Chagla and Chakrabarti had teamed up with a professor at the University of British Columbia to address the issue that frustrates many infectious disease doctors: the perception that it's easy to get infected with Covid outside.

The piece, published in the *Toronto Star* in mid-April, was titled "Why We Need to Change the Narrative on Outdoor Transmission." Here's an excerpt:

> *Each of us can also resist the temptation to shame-and-blame people gathering outdoors. Almost every weekend last summer, social media was filled with tut-tutting at pictures of those congregating outdoors, generally in fairly small groups. Those remonstrations have ramped up again now that spring has arrived. What if we turned the narrative on its head and thanked those people for meeting outdoors rather than indoors? Shaming people for gathering outdoors is likely to drive them indoors, where COVID transmission is far more likely. Let's use communication to encourage less risky behaviour rather than stigmatize it.*

Chagla says, "That one seemed to generate a lot of dis-taste, and I don't understand why. Again, we really tried to frame it as this is something that is reasonable and rational, and people can do and feel normal, and really describe the evidence behind it. We gotta stop shaming people for being outside. I thought that was a message we got rid of last year after the Trinity Bellwoods issue [when pictures of people socializing in the Toronto park were posted on social and mainstream media with critical comments]. But again, a lot of people said, 'You don't know about variants,' 'We don't want kids around there,' 'All these people are close together.'"

What was more difficult to understand than the public reaction was what the Ontario government did. "It was wild because literally four days after that, [Ontario's premier] Doug Ford and the PC Party actually shut down playgrounds and parks. This didn't make any sense. That was the com-plete opposite we were trying to achieve with this article."

The provincial government did quickly change course on its playground policy, and who knows to what extent the *Toronto Star* commentary influenced them or members of the public. But whatever benefits came from the op-eds, Chagla had learned there would be criticism. "Every one of these op-eds was met by resistance by some people. Typically our op-eds have been reasonable in trying to bridge the gap between both sides, but obviously that means there are people on both sides who don't agree with those opinions, and so be it. However, they've been a very therapeutic way to get our message across and put something in a longer form that people can read."

"Therapeutic" is likely not the word Chagla and Chakrabarti would use to describe one of their most widely read pieces. At least, it probably didn't seem therapeutic in the first few days after it was published. I think it's one of the most interesting examples of the motivation infectious disease doctors have to get their message out, as well as the risks they take. In this case, that risk was to their own reputations and their working relationships with some colleagues.

Perhaps you saw the commentary, titled "South Asians Play a Part in COVID-19 Transmission and We Need to Acknowledge It," in the *Toronto Star* on a Sunday in mid-November 2020. Or maybe, like me, you read it online as it ricocheted around the internet, shared, forwarded and commented on by lots of people. Chagla and Chakrabarti wrote it with Tajinder Kaura, an emergency medicine physician. Here's how it began:

> *Canadian society is an interwoven matrix of multiculturalism that contributes to the strength of our nation. The South Asian community comprises a significant part of this rich heterogeneity. Today, we write to you both as physicians, and also members of this vibrant community.*

They cited statistics that showed members of the South Asian community were getting Covid at higher rates than the general Canadian population and were more likely to die from the virus. The piece went on to list various factors (for example, multi-generational households and the preponderance of front line workers who couldn't work from home). But what drew angry criticism was the focus of the article: how the culture of social gatherings in the South Asian community was increasing Covid transmission.

> *One such theme is hospitality to others, no matter what background or creed. A guest leaving your house on an empty stomach is considered a travesty, and results in long meals and conversation.*

And so, among the recommendations:

> *Indoor gatherings of individuals outside of our direct household must be temporarily stopped in order to limit spread—particularly with large celebrations, such as Diwali, upcoming.*
> *We need to be creative with outdoor spaces, trying to allow for some in person interaction while minimizing risk.*

Their motivation in making that point, says Chakrabarti, was simple. They were deeply worried. "We were seeing people have large weddings, people going to India and coming back. I was seeing it on the ground. Oh my God, the ICU was filled with South Asian people, and the same thing was happening in England and Surrey [British Columbia]. People crammed into living rooms singing—these things were leading to outbreaks."

Chagla adds, "We both recognized the problem is not all cultural, though that was part of it. I had been working with my own religious community to keep our congregate settings safe and really get people to heed advice." But as case and ICU numbers in the South Asian community kept rising, the doctors felt they had to get the message out.

Chagla says their co-writer, Dr. Kaura, "was working at assessment centres, seeing 20 to 30 per cent positives of people walking in, rates exploding, hospitals filling up. We keep tiptoeing around this problem but we weren't talking about it." Chagla says he, Chakrabarti and Kaura realized "we need to inspire change. We need to talk to our own people, to say the cultural norms don't apply here. We all understood Indian people are very bright, and generally they want to follow public health rules, but there was a lot of pointing to say, 'This is that person's problem. My relatives are safe, my friends and family are safe, and therefore we're not going to be at risk for Covid.'"

The op-ed didn't only focus on culture and lifestyle. Chakrabarti points out, "We all know there are certain structural factors that lead to problems, hitting people with lower income, living with larger families." And so they wrote:

> *Understanding the cultural contexts that are unique to our population, such as multi-generational families, public-facing occupations, poor English literacy, and densely populated communities, allows for individualized planning that benefits society as a whole . . .*

> *Encouraging healthy workplaces, particularly*
> *reinforcing indoor masking and avoidance of pro-*
> *longed close contact is paramount.*

But Chakrabarti says there was an unwillingness to address the extent to which personal choices could reduce infection rates. He says, "One thing we thought was really being lost in the narrative was people assume racialized people are poor," and thus not able to control all the risk factors. And it was clear to him that a lot of people didn't want to address the disproportionate rates of Covid infection in the community. "Our goal was to get that message out there, understanding there was a structural issue that people can't control, but there are certain things we can do for risk mitigation. We thought we could talk to the group about that because we're from the group."

Chagla adds, "We needed to be explicit. We need to tell this story—no one is going to tell it other than people of that background—and be very honest and abrupt and explicit about it. And it was a reasonable article to write. We had very good evidence from Toronto, from StatsCan, really talking about the impacts on our community."

A few days later the *Toronto Star* published a second op-ed by another three members of the South Asian community, including two doctors. It criticized the earlier commentary, saying it

> *blamed and shamed our South Asian commun-*
> *ities for the spike in cases as a result of weddings*

*and religious celebrations like Diwali and Bandi
Chhor Divas.*

*But what's missing from the real story? The
stark, staggering inequities faced by this population
were largely dismissed among the cultural stereotypes
reinforced in this article.*

A lot of the reaction on Twitter was equally harsh. A
Toronto-area doctor wrote:

> Continually blaming Brown people in
> Brampton for rising #COVID19 cases is
> unnerving & racist.
> Instead of learning how people's
> vulnerabilities are guided by their
> circumstances (multi-generational
> households, poverty & employment), we
> lay blame.
> How is this constructive?

Another doctor, this one in British Columbia, tweeted:

> Same problem being seen in Surrey, BC.
> It is much easier for people to blame
> South Asians, rather than exploring the
> root cause, appreciating the struggle of
> disproportionately affected communities
> and offering relief + support in this
> difficult time.

Chakrabarti responds, "We had to say something. We got a lot of love for it and we got a lot of hate too. I'm fine with it because this led to the formation of the South Asian Covid task force, and we were really able to get messaging out to the South Asian community in Brampton. They've opened up testing centres, vaccine clinics. It really did end up doing a lot of good, but a lot of people didn't want to touch the topic because it's almost like if you talk about someone with brown skin, it's automatically a bad thing. Of course there are issues [the South Asian community] can't control, but there are things we can control, and I think it made a difference."

He continues, "It's hard to forget all the people who sent nasty tweets. I was quite disappointed because there were a couple of people that I knew, who know who I am, who know I'm not trying to slam dunk on brown people's heads. That is what disappointed me the most. I knew there were people who would never see this message eye to eye, but I think the disappointing thing was a couple of friends of mine, people I'd known from med school, I'd known professionally from university, and I thought, you know, 'I'm not this person you're publicly accusing me of being,' so it's kind of disappointing. But the vast majority of people who knew me, including many Indians, said, 'Thank you for saying this. We know it's been happening and no one can talk about it.'"

Chagla adds, "I think some people didn't realize we were there in the community, talking to people, dealing with people, working with people, seeing this first-hand. We were getting these stories. But somehow, some people felt we were trespassers and trying to invoke a more racial presentation of Indians, which was not our intent whatsoever.

"Being trusted voices was the point, and there was a lot of negative feedback in social media and in traditional media. People accused us of not talking enough about front-facing workers and support for poverty, and we did talk about that. It's not like it wasn't mentioned in that article. It was there. But we did also include culture. Gatherings are part of our culture as with every other person who has to deal with it.

"At the end of the day, all of us were a little bit taken aback but realized this wasn't going to be the perfect article. People will always complain about something. At the end of the day there was a lot of progress."

It has been fascinating to watch the ID doctors manage their direct communication with the public, from Saxinger's Twitter blend of the personal and professional to Bogoch's all news, all the time. Neither approach is better than the other, just different.

Equally interesting is how they've dealt with the backlash. Whether it's Susy Hota stepping away from Twitter rather than getting into an unseemly public spat with other scientists, or Chakrabarti and Chagla continuing to produce op-eds, undeterred by the bruising criticism of their piece on Covid in the South Asian community.

That commentary is an illustration of the sense of duty they feel to reach beyond the hospital setting and try to change behaviours in a way that will reduce transmission. Months later, Chagla says, "If it took us putting our reputations on the line and getting battered in the media, then so be it. At the end of the day it achieved what it needed to achieve, and Sumon and Taj and I are very proud of what we put out and we'd do it again in a heartbeat."

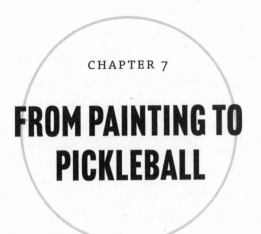

CHAPTER 7

FROM PAINTING TO PICKLEBALL

WHEN I CONNECT WITH EACH OF THESE DOCTORS ON the phone, I am mindful of the many demands on their time. I know there are questions I need to get to—finding out about their background, hearing what it was like early in the pandemic and, of course, asking how they deal with the media. But toward the end of the phone calls, there are always a few extra minutes.

That doesn't often happen when I do interviews. So I enjoy the privilege of indulging myself by asking questions that aren't essential but that I've been really curious about. Like, "Lisa Barrett, what's up with that huge painting behind you?"

To my relief, she answers with a laugh. It's not the first time she's been asked about it. Before the pandemic, Barrett would do media interviews from work. But when the demands increased, she ran into the challenge facing many of us, whether it's for work or an interview on the news: where do you set up a makeshift home studio? Barrett settled on the one place in her apartment with fixed lighting, no shadows. She says, "That's where I've sat for thousands of Zoom meetings and many many media interviews."

She wasn't looking to showcase the large canvas. It just turned out that way. "It was the best thing to put behind me. Honest to goodness, it was just truly fortuitous. It's a good thing some people at least like it, because I didn't have anything else to put there."

I ask Barrett if the painting has become well known in Atlantic Canada. "Oh, hands down!" she says with a laugh. "I've gotten cards, letters, emails. Steve Murphy [the legendary anchor of CTV's supper-hour news in the Maritimes] regularly forwards me the usual plethora of fan mail and says, 'Can't you just give me the name of the artist so we can send it out for you?' And I say, 'Yes, absolutely, go for it.'"

Barrett pauses for a moment. "Of course, it's not the best background because it's too much and it's too close and it's blah blah blah [that's a direct quote]. But you know what? It's certainly become iconic around these parts, that's for sure."

She points out in this case, at least, fame does not come at a high cost. "I bought it in grad school when, you know, you don't have a lot of money, and clearly I haven't had time to buy real art. It's from one of those online stores that prints oversize canvases, which I love. Not local, not expensive, but it appeals to me in many ways. I'm very grateful to the artist of that painting."

There are different ways to spruce up a blank background. As I mentioned earlier, Lynora Saxinger uses a plant, which, when she catches a glimpse of it on TV, sometimes leads her to fret it hasn't been watered enough.

The plant is not anything more meaningful than a plant. I say that because of Sumon Chakrabarti's TV backdrop. He is always perfectly framed between two guitar cases. I thought maybe this was just a random background in a spare bedroom, but I was wrong. It is carefully curated. Chakrabarti describes the guitars as "a cornerstone of my life. One of them is a Gibson Les Paul electric that I got for myself after I finished my training in 2010. It's the same one as Slash in Guns N' Roses uses. I've always wanted to be him. [An excellent question, by the way, for the Infectious Disease Doctors edition of Trivial Pursuit.] And the other one was a fortieth-birthday present from my wife. It's a Martin acoustic. It's emblematic of who I am. I grew up with guitars and music. Been in bands. It's a piece of me on the screen for people to see."

As we chat about his background, Chakrabarti says he feels very comfortable on the air now, but admits that early on, quite understandably, he was nervous (an admission I'm not sure everyone would make). "I could actually feel my heart starting to beat faster, and that would affect how I was speaking. If that happens now, it doesn't really affect me."

Zain Chagla has been able to perfect his on-air work courtesy of a high-powered in-house consultant. "My wife is in digital marketing, so she looked at my interviews and critiqued that part, and hammered down the language and the mannerisms and the things that can hinder some of the messaging, but also worked with me making sure I was conveying the fundamental message of what you want to say without the audience being redirected. I thank her for that. That is certainly one of the things that helped in the first month where I was a bit nervous doing all of this."

He jokes (at least, I think he's joking), "These were awkward, awkward conversations, but obviously coming from someone I know has my best interests and wants me to be a better communicator, probably personally, and in the media. She'd point out places I was using filler words, using particular mannerisms, if I wasn't getting to the point. My parents would watch and say, 'You did great.' That's not really feedback. But she coaches executives so I welcomed all that experience."

Another surprising discovery from my research was "The Lisa Barrett Media Archive," my title for a collection of her interviews, lovingly compiled and curated by her mother. Barrett says that every time she books an interview, it's on a Google calendar that her parents can see as well. "There is—I will not lie to you—a tape or audio recording of almost every single interview I've done since last March. It's sweet of them." She adds—perhaps to ensure I don't think of her parents as obsessive fans of their daughter—"They see this media work as part of public service, and that's always been important. You should contribute and this is a good way to contribute."

One of the pieces of tape they've collected is also preserved on YouTube. The interview from CPAC, the Canadian Public Affairs Channel, gives an example of how deftly Barrett handles on-air surprises.

During an episode of *PrimeTime Politics* in April 2021, host Peter Van Dusen is speaking to Barrett about vaccine side effects. The first question is simple enough: how concerned is she about side effects from the Johnson & Johnson vaccine. She gives a detailed answer, citing evidence of the very rare possibility of blood clots, and finishes with "Do I think that makes it a globally unsafe vaccine? No. Do I think it's the right thing to pause? Yes."

But then, the twist. Van Dusen looks down at a piece of paper, a statement from the Public Health Agency of Canada, that apparently has just been handed to him. As a viewer, you wonder what this breaking development is. I'm fascinated to watch Barrett's face, which remains on the screen as she hears for the first time what Van Dusen is reading.

The news is the first reported Canadian case of a person getting serious blood clots linked to the AstraZeneca vaccine. Van Dusen asks, "should that change our thinking at all, because now we've heard about these other incidents in Europe, and now, looks like we might have a case?" It's a completely fair but challenging question, especially to news that has just broken.

Almost without a pause, Barrett answers. "Well, the European medical agency had been further investigating these low platelets, special blood clots, um, further and it really wasn't able to exclude a link, though very very rare, with the AstraZeneca . . . So it's not unexpected that after we had given some doses that we might see a case." As someone who watches and studies a lot of interviews, I am impressed by how clear her answer is as she goes through what is known about clots related to the vaccine, and concludes with "I hope this person is doing well, and it will be important to see how old this person is, and what the other circumstances were around their health status."

That was how it looked on the air. Six weeks later I ask her if she remembers that moment—she does—and what she was thinking as she heard the new information. "The first thing that goes through your head is 'Oh shit.'" I assume she means she wasn't expecting that surprise question. But I'm wrong. "My first thought was I knew [a case of VITT—vaccine-induced clots] was going to show up eventually, and I was concerned for the patient."

That was her first thought. Then, still listening to the question, she was thinking about the opinion on the AstraZeneca vaccine that she had been sharing in earlier interviews. While most public health officials and many doctors simply said, "Take the first vaccine offered to you," Barrett says her guidance had been slightly different. "On any vaccine I've always said, 'Balance your risk and benefit.' If you're in a place that has zero Covid, and you have the option of waiting for a bit, you can, right? If you're worried about this, you should have informed decision making.

"So what was I thinking? I felt terrible for the person, but also, to be honest, I'm glad I've been tempered in the way I've approached it. It never felt quite right to me to tell people you have to get the first thing that comes to you, because it didn't give people licence to make choices that they might need or want to make. And then the third thing was, how do you make sense of this for people without taking away from the true benefits of the vaccine?" A lot to think about during a short, surprising question.

Susy Hota was involved in a similar moment, on CBC News Network, in the very early days of Covid. I didn't realize what was going on behind the scenes until Hota told me, more than a year later.

It was Saturday, January 25, 2020, and Hota was heading to the CBC Broadcast Centre. "I didn't know the exact topic, and while I was on the streetcar I got a call from the CEO of my hospital." She was told Ontario's first patient with Covid was in a Toronto-area hospital. "That's a moment I won't forget. It was a milestone event. Breaking news, right on my phone on the streetcar. I remember thinking, 'I'm going to need some details on what's happened.'"

But when she arrived at the Broadcast Centre, the news still wasn't out. She sat down with host Natasha Fatah just after 5 p.m., eastern time. The interview was long, relaxed and, for the first five minutes, exactly what you'd expect at that point in the story. What are the symptoms of Covid? How concerned should we be in Canada?

As Hota sat in the chair, news was happening. Fatah said, "While you were giving that last answer, I was handed a piece of paper with some information I want to share with you. We are getting information that the Ontario Chief Medical Officer of Health is going to be making an announcement, that's at 5:30 p.m., eastern time, so we're going to be watching for that."

Only now, watching that tape, do I realize how tricky a situation that was. Hota was pretty sure what that announcement was going to be, but it wasn't her role to disclose the information. She didn't want to say what it likely was, but at the same time she didn't want to say she had no idea. So she was careful, deftly explaining who would likely be at that news conference with the health officer and that—technically true—we didn't know the topic of the news conference.

Fatah, of course, had no idea what Hota knew, and she asked a pretty smart question. "What are you going to be listening for at that press conference?"

Hota's equally smart answer: "I would like to hear details on what's going on and what their take is."

Later, she explains to me that, as a doctor, she's accustomed to keeping information confidential, although this situation was different from what she was used to. "It's so important to be careful what you say when you know something that hasn't been made public, and you know it from a different source. I'm always very cautious about that kind of thing. So at least I had been warned and thought through how I could deal with it. But it's always uncomfortable. You feel in a way you're being dishonest, but at the same time it's not my place to be speaking about it. There's a whole reason there's a press conference with the right people there to talk about it. To be honest, it was one of the most interesting timings of an interview."

I'm not sure how our guests on TV feel, but as a broadcaster and a viewer, I love the unpredictability of unscripted, live television. You can be on the air at the moment new information is coming in, or as you cover the chaos of a riot or rising flood waters. These are the important, life-changing stories that are often noted and replayed on the anniversaries and on awards nights.

But I hope that somewhere, someone in Canadian broadcasting is also noting another category of live moments, the more whimsical ones. Greg Ross, for example, spotting Drake during CBC's live coverage of the Toronto Raptors' NBA championship parade in June 2019, tossing him a wireless mike, getting a comment from the music superstar and then, when Drake tosses it back, continuing his coverage without missing a beat. Or one of my favourite pandemic media moments: what should forever be referred to as "The Pickleball Incident," starring Isaac Bogoch and his wife, Linda.

Bogoch says, "I feel like I'm the butt of every pickleball joke, and it's hysterical. I love just how whenever there's a pickleball reference, Covid or non-Covid, someone will shout out, 'Hey, Bogoch, pickleball!'"

Again, Natasha Fatah was the host on CBC News Network for another long, topical interview in late October 2020. Among her questions: What should we make of a surge of cases two weeks after Thanksgiving? And what were the doctor's thoughts on a pilot program in Alberta to test people coming in from the United States? Then Fatah reads an email from a viewer: "Is it advisable to play pickleball indoors at a recreation centre?" Bogoch laughs and says he has no idea what pickleball is. Then he answers in a more general way, saying that, in Toronto, it would probably be discouraged to play a sport indoors with people not in your household. After some light banter about what pickleball is, they move on to the next viewer question, asking whether Covid can be transmitted through a building's ventilation system.

You can't tell by watching the video, but Bogoch can hear something in the background. "I thought it was my kids scratching on the door. I don't know if it comes out in the interviews, but sometimes my kids are pounding on that door, yelling, 'Dad, let's go outside.' I just thought it was them and I try not to get distracted. But I'm watching the screen—I can see myself on the screen and can see movement behind me. We have the flimsiest of locks on the door. It's meant to keep toddlers out, but my kids are older than that. I always thought, 'One day the kids are going to break into the room.'"

The door behind him swings open, and Bogoch says, "Oh, we've got a neighbour," then turns around and says, "We're on live TV."

Later he tells me, "I see it's my wife, and I'm shocked. I don't remember what I said, it's like 'Someone's here.' She hands me the pickleball racquets. I wanted to have some composure. I tried to answer the question, but Natasha was hysterical." And by hysterical, he means doubled over laughing.

Bogoch, also laughing in the interview, says, "Apparently we have pickleball," and Fatah, as if they've done this routine a million times before, says he clearly is not the main player in the house. Then, after a pause, he resumes his answer about airborne transmission in mid-sentence.

When Fatah posted the clip on Twitter, it got thousands of views and likes and lots of approving comments

("That made my day," "Dr. Bogoch's wife wins 'Best Canadian Cameo By A Spouse,'" "Fantastic, fun interview"). Even some of his fellow ID docs weighed in, including Lynora Saxinger ("I had my dog Muppet break in on a live Q & A with Carole McNeil. It's good fun and nice to acknowledge everyone's essential humanity") and Sumon Chakrabarti ("Isaac, if you don't end up liking pickleball, come and play tennis with me. Naturally physically distanced and way more exciting").

Bogoch's assessment? In his lighthearted tone, he says this won't be happening again. "On the one hand, I thought it was funny. On the other hand, that is a one-time event. You don't want people to get into the habit of walking into the interview because, quite frankly, it's work. It's not an official job, but it's something I take seriously. It would be less hysterical if it were a common event. I don't want to be the news. I'm happy to talk about it. I don't want to be it."

Speaking of talking about the news, I ask each of the doctors to reflect on their time in the media spotlight. As I have learned in our conversations, they are thoughtful and analytical, and that's reflected in their comments.

Zain Chagla has a theory on why ID docs have done so well speaking publicly during the pandemic. "I think there's something to be said about someone who can understand the science and has to be accountable to patients on a day-to-day basis. You see people like Isaac, Sumon, Lynora. They try to balance that. Again, to talk to a patient takes a huge amount of ability to process knowledge and put it in terms that people understand and be pragmatic, right?"

In terms of pragmatism, he offers an example. "I would love to have everyone wear N95 masks all day and have perfectly ventilated settings, but there's also the art of the possible and what people can do versus what should be done in that situation. That is sometimes missed in all of this."

So being pragmatic is important. But the ever-present challenge for anyone who appears in the media is balancing the reach (in some cases a single interview will be seen by more than a million people) with the constraints of time, format and editing.

Sumon Chakrabarti says, "Doing the ninety-second thing can be tough," but perhaps more challenging is when a reporter or someone on social media only uses a short excerpt, in or out of context. He says that "the sensational bites will often get the most press." But, notably, that hasn't deterred him or the others from answering the calls and trying to convey complex science to an anxious and sometimes highly partisan audience.

Chagla points out another continuing challenge: trying to reach people who just fundamentally disagree with what you say, even if it's correct. "It's tough, right? You want to quote evidence, you want to be reasonable. I spend time listening to people on both sides of the spectrum. It gives me a better understanding that you're never going to make everyone happy. This may be a scientific issue, but there is a political spectrum that applies to this for some people. All you can do is try to follow the science, be reasonable, but also understand it's much more than just facts and figures. It is literally a pandemic that affects everyone, and I think that affects the way people understand the evidence. A lot gets lost in the translation."

You might be wondering how a busy doctor gets to hear a wide range of voices. For Chagla, one source is listening to talk radio during his commute. "I'm at work all day dealing with pandemic issues, modelling, public health. Then I get in the car and I listen to radio about pandemic issues, modelling, public health." He laughs. "It's a nice barometer of what's going on—what people are thinking about this, average everyday people."

He also pays attention to other professionals to see "how other people are approaching this communication, what they're feeling as different clinicians. That's a learning experience in terms of how, for example, you actually communicate risk appropriately. How do you resonate with people, as opposed to just yelling and screaming expletives? Like it or not, you have become a public communicator. If you have a good message, you want to make sure it resonates, as opposed to being the contrarian who's always interviewed because their opinion is one-sided and you know exactly what's going to happen."

Without prompting, he cites BC's Provincial Health Officer, Dr. Bonnie Henry, as "the epitome of public health communication. I can't say she's always been right about everything, but she puts it out there in a way that's reassuring, non-alarming, makes the public a stakeholder, really tries to convey and distill reasonable points, and tries to present balance from a scientific standpoint rather than from a personal feeling standpoint. The public is a stakeholder on this.

They're reading voraciously too. They're confused by much of what's going on. And you really need to distill things down into language that's appropriate but also accurate. You need to recognize your own biases in the way you communicate, and I'm shocked every day by my friends and colleagues, who I thought were much more reasonable and much more intelligent and able to recognize their own biases, who are clearly playing their own biases out on the air and in the public and on social media."

As Chagla continues, it's clear he has given this issue a lot of thought. "I think it's important to have the humility to be wrong. There are things I've been wrong on in this pandemic, and you need the ability to pivot, to live with some uncertainty, the ability to not make definitive statements but try to encourage responsible statements as appropriate.

"Getting to the point, speaking clearly, using salient examples, but not getting lost in the emotion of what's happening as well. There have been moments where I've been frustrated and let that out on the air, but I don't think it resonates with people to see a pissed-off doctor."

We are speaking during the surge of the third wave, when some people seem to be flouting the rules and some governments appear to be ignoring the advice of their own scientists. When I laugh at Chagla's reference to an angry doctor, he gently pushes back. "It's true. We're seeing it more and more. The person who's lost their business, or missing their parents or friends and family, doesn't want to see a pissed-off doctor. They don't want to see someone yelling, 'You're killing everyone.' Things need to be done, for sure, but that's not a responsible way to convey it. Again, Dr. Henry is the epitome of this."

Srinivas Murthy has also given a lot of thought to his media role during the pandemic. I ask what he's learned. "It's important to acknowledge where your expertise is, but also acknowledging where your expertise is not, and being very careful not to trespass beyond what you think you know. I read things and I keep up to date on things, but I don't claim expertise on all things coronavirus related, nor should any one individual.

"Knowing where those boundaries are is crucial. I think at the beginning, when no one knew anything, I felt more comfortable talking more broadly about how the world was and what we could do. Now, with so much information out there, I'm trying to keep some guardrails on things I will talk about and things I won't talk about. I've learned over-stepping your knowledge set leads to misinterpretation and challenges.

"Second, the thrill of people listening to you, it's part of your job as a doctor. But when that's amplified with media appearances, appearing on the national news and so on, there is some sort of joy in that. You feel honoured to be part of that communication with the public, but at the same time, that can very quickly turn to amplifying your own ego and make you more confident in your skill set and expertise, even if you don't have that expertise."

Murthy says one challenge for him was deciding what to do when he was asked before an interview to discuss a Covid topic he didn't know a lot about. He didn't like the idea of quickly reading up on it and then relaying the information. "I felt uncomfortable because I should know things as an expert that reflect why people are asking, and I shouldn't have to scramble to learn something to communicate to reporters."

When I press him on this, he does acknowledge he wouldn't simply be repeating what he'd read but applying his specialist's lens. And it is something he would do. "When you're asking me about airborne transmission and then following up with school policy and follow up with disease treatment, I can speak intensely about a couple of those things and loosely about the third, but I probably have the foundational knowledge to communicate to the public in a clear way without that specific expertise."

I am interviewing Murthy by phone on a beautiful spring day, as case counts are concerningly high in British Columbia and public health officials are warning people to remain vigilant. This set of circumstances reminds Murthy of the careful messaging that experts need to convey. He uses an example that will be familiar to many readers.

"Risk communication is a difficult thing, and you need people who have experience communicating risk to individuals to get that message out there. When you talk about the balance of risks right now with widespread disease transmission—which will likely continue for the next few weeks with blue skies and cherry blossoms—to keep people sane within this next few weeks, to embrace things that get them joy is a useful intervention. Balancing risk and balancing benefits is part of every conversation I have with patients all the time, and trying to communicate that to the public in tweets or in news clips is always difficult because it's going to be nuanced and it's going to be challenging to convey. But at least trying to get people through this very difficult situation is important.

"I know that approach has been criticized by some who feel we need to be, quote, draconian slash lock things down and stay at home and so on, and I think you can do both. You can be strict about the situations that lead to challenges for transmission but also allow some people to have some liberty and joy in their lives, which I think they need right now."

I tell Murthy that when I listen to ID docs, it seems like they are skilled at balancing the scientific evidence and the art of human nature and communication. He agrees. "I think we all recognize in the biomedical science space only a part of this outbreak response is going to have science data. So much of how we're going to get through this is not science but more policy and more social science. Obviously I'm not an expert in that, but we are experts in talking to people and communicating risk and harm and making hard decisions, and with that expertise we can apply the science and allow it to be an art."

This is what Chagla is referring to when he says that talking to so many patients over the years helps develop the "ability to process knowledge and put it in terms that people understand." He tells me about a podcast he listens to featuring Monica Gandhi, a US infectious disease doctor. "There are a lot of people being called by the media, but very few of them are people who have to walk the walk and talk the talk on a daily basis, and they're the ones who are able to distill down the black and white into things that are reasonable as opposed to things that are important to adhere to. She talked about this and said, in the pandemic, physicians didn't have the ability to work from home. They were still seeing patients, they were in the thick of things and they were exposing their families to risk. But being a physician also gives you that shared decision-making, risk-mitigation, harm-reduction lens that you use for patients.

"People who are able to communicate the science properly probably have a background of not only the science but are living it in their day-to-day lives. They're forced to be out there, forced to wear masks all day, forced to talk to patients about risk, and that is an unspoken skill that distinguished them from those who haven't had that practical experience."

Infectious disease doctors also have to calculate and communicate risk for cross-sections of society and for circumstances most of us might not think about. Chakrabarti gives the example of a decision in Ontario early in the pandemic to shut down strip bars. "There was a lot of moralizing about the Covid response. I know strip bars are not everyone's thing, but it is a legal business. But they were shuttered way early in the pandemic and everyone was, like, 'Yeah, okay, shut them.' The thing is, I've seen women who were working in some of these establishments. I saw them before the pandemic, and they ended up going into the sex trade. There was disease, violence."

Chagla says he and his colleagues often have an insight that may not be clear to politicians and members of the public. "It was easy for people to kick someone to the side and not realize the unintended consequences."

At the end of my last interview with Bogoch, I ask him if he has anything he wants to talk about. "I have found my interactions with the media so pleasant and so good," he replies, "and even when they're asking hard questions, everyone has been polite, professional and genuinely interested in getting to the root of the problem—scientific or policy. They've always been respectful of my time. It's just been very very good interactions with the media.

"And as you know, I'm not shying away. I will talk to anyone. That means left-of-centre media, right-of-centre, anyone in between. I'll stick to my story and I'll stick to what needs to be said, regardless of who I'm speaking with, but mostly—I don't want to jinx anything—but to date I really haven't had a bad experience. I find the media very professional.

"Just like in medicine, where we have redeployment—in the media, people who are sports reporters and parliamentary reporters are now spending a lot of time focusing on COVID-19, and they are generally very eager to get it right and very eager to get the technical aspects correct, scientific jargon translated to plain English. I think relative to the rest of the world, Canadian media covered this really really well, largely in a very fair manner. And my personal interactions, and there have probably been over a thousand, have all been very good."

Lynora Saxinger has also had good experiences with reporters. "One of the pluses of dealing with the more traditional media role has been—and this was unexpected—I didn't realize how having trained communicators and questioners interact with you would help you think about things better. Usually you get down your sciency path, and in all of the discussions I've had, having people interrogate from different angles has sometimes proven really important for me in terms of getting into how people perceive things, and even how I'm thinking about them and whether I should broaden out what I'm thinking. That process of sensemaking for the public can sometimes be sensemaking for me, because it makes me handle that information differently. Being able to explain things in a suitable way sometimes helps me distill it as well.

"And I've come to appreciate the art of communication more. There is journalistic art, and I think it can be almost magical how I can say something that sounds super boring, and then someone writes it up and it sounds really good, and I'm, like, 'What? You guys are great!'" She laughs. "I think there's some kind of interesting synergy there. As a takeaway and going forward, I'd like to have the leisure to think about that some more. What is that space? What is that synergy for a content expert and a communication journalism expert, because I think it's going to stay important even after the pandemic. That's been cool.

"And it is gratifying to think you might be able to help shape how things are evolving—with good intentions, obviously. Not with an evil laugh or anything. I think there's a certain potency to that, which I think people should try not to get drunk on and should handle responsibly."

Saxinger points out one of the most important aspects of having independent experts from across the country weigh in on policies developed by public health doctors and enacted by governments: "I actually do think having a diversity of voices to talk about things, and trying to really have a principled take on trying to help the public discourse—not potshots—and try to help break down the silos is really important. And that's been important all the way along. These silos, almost tribal groups, are both within science and within the public. Trying to find a space between that, where you can have a sensible discussion, is something where the traditional media has a huge edge over social media platforms. But it's also a place where people aren't going as much as they used to, and I think that's a really big loss."

She remembers a much different time when it came to the influence of the mainstream media. "It used to be that people of various backgrounds would watch the same news and interpret it and discuss it. They were actually starting from that place in the middle, where now everyone is getting their media pre-filtered through some pretty extreme lenses sometimes. So they're not starting from that common place, and you can really see it and feel it. It's a really big threat, not just for public health—for society at large."

Lisa Barrett also says her many interactions with the media have been respectful and productive. "The media stuff for me has been a privilege, and I've gotten as much out of it—and the ability to feel that I'm contributing—as much as anyone has gotten from me."

But she concedes not every expert guest feels that way. She tells me about a colleague "who's taken a bit of a beating [in news coverage], is really uncomfortable with the media, and I said to her, 'Why? They're people. The goal here for all of us is the same, I think.' But people don't always perceive it as the same, and they don't feel they have the ability to frame things well, in which case maybe you shouldn't do a lot of it."

Perhaps part of Barrett's success is her ability to handle the unexpected. We saw it in the CPAC interview, where she handled that surprise question smoothly. She also revealed one of her "tricks," which she uses sometimes to shift an interview where she'd like it to go: "I will often say, 'That's the question you asked, but if I were to ask the question, I would ask a slightly different one.'" (I'm not sure my fellow journalists want to encourage this behaviour by expert guests, but I feel obliged to include Dr. Barrett's subversive technique.)

After eighteen months of interviews in French and English, Fatima Kakkar says, "It's really struck me how we're not trained for media work, but how important it is in this pandemic to speak clearly, and how much of an influence it has on people's decisions." We are speaking the same week the National Advisory Council on Immunization (NACI) said there could be circumstances where someone might choose not to have the AstraZeneca vaccine, and might wait for one of the mRNA vaccines (Pfizer or Moderna) instead. NACI said people should consider their tolerance for the low risk of getting blood clots against their risk of getting Covid. The council's suggestion that AstraZeneca might not be the "preferred vaccine" created instant controversy. Kakkar says, "All I have to do is think back to yesterday's NACI debacle and—I can't blame them, I know them, they're all physicians and they've been doing research and science their whole lives. But they're not used to picking their words with such precision, and you realize these words have such an impact."

Kakkar has already noted how mindful she is of the careful scrutiny of French-language interviews, and she says, "We've never been in this position before, but it's been one of those eye-opening things where I've realized the impact of our words. Just being a physician, being an ID expert, your words are taken very seriously, so I have to think about how I say things and what I say."

Reflecting on her own position as a pediatrician working in a hospital, who is now being asked about the safety of keeping kids in school, she concludes, "I think there is a sense of duty. At some point when it came to kids and Covid, I realized I know this better than most people, and people want this information. They need to know this, so it was that sense of duty. And I think that's our nature as physicians, and we didn't really question our obligation. We do things in the line of duty, and afterwards we think about it and say, 'What's the risk assessment?' We do what we have to do, and when you're the content expert in a specific area, you feel obliged to speak up. It was important to speak up about the data and calm people down and reassure them. And I figured if I didn't do it, maybe someone else who knew less or was less directly involved with kids might speak up and not necessarily have that same information."

I'll finish this section with Susy Hota. As a hospital executive who is also an infectious disease doctor working in the biggest media market in the country, she accepted all interview requests in the early weeks of the pandemic. Her assessment of how that went: "I've been very impressed with how all the media outlets I've worked with have tried to cover things as fairly as possible. It's not an easy task, I know that. There's so much coming from so many directions, and so many opinions. Some issues have become very hot-button and polarized, and it's hard to sort through all that. If things had been different, that may have swayed me to not engage with that outlet. But it hasn't happened. The interviewers, the reporters, the producers, everyone has been so respectful and trying very hard."

It's not that Hota is reluctant to call out unfair reporting. She tells me, "I did a fair amount of media during the H1N1 pandemic—the pandemic that was forgotten—and during that time I did have a few interviews that didn't go so well and where I felt very confronted. There were attempts to catch me saying things I shouldn't be saying, and it did make it a lot harder because that wall that I had, being very cautious about what I would share, was definitely higher up. Now I feel much more comfortable talking to reporters."

During the Covid pandemic, she says, "I haven't come across a situation where I feel I've been misquoted or I've been put into a situation deliberately where I'm going to say something that's going to cause harm to myself or is going to be misconstrued. People have tried to clarify, and I've had reporters come back and say, 'I just want to make sure I got the right essence of what you're trying to say,' and that makes all the difference to those of us who put ourselves out there."

I didn't ask any of the doctors about media coverage. But when I hear their comments, I realize it's not just the infectious disease doctors who made the coverage of Covid different. It was the approach of journalists as well. And while that comment may seem self-serving, this is not about *The National* or CBC but, rather, every major news organization in Canada. People like Global's Keith Baldrey, the *Globe and Mail's* Andre Picard, podcaster Ryan Jespersen and so many others have covered this story with a high degree of care.

This is a very competitive business. We are always trying to outdo other media outlets and sometimes our own colleagues. And no story was bigger than Covid. But somehow the competition did not turn into "gotcha" journalism, juicy soundbites or provocative headlines. The coverage was extensive, careful and as complete as we could make it. And the infectious disease doctors helped us achieve that.

CHAPTER 8

RETURN TO ANONYMITY

A SENSE OF DUTY. THAT'S HOW FATIMA KAKKAR DESCRIBED why she felt compelled to step into the media spotlight during the pandemic. And while not every doctor in the book used that word, it's clear they felt it too.

Usually when someone I want to interview mentions the word "duty," they're referring to a technical, legal requirement—their fiduciary duty or duty to a client, for example—and it's usually cited as a reason why they can't speak to me or say much. But for the infectious disease doctors, this duty was personal. There's nothing in their employment contract or in the rules of the College of Physicians and Surgeons that requires doing hundreds of hours of media interviews. But they saw it as an extension of the guidance and reassurance they were providing friends and colleagues and patients, amplified by mass media.

When I set out to write this book, I wanted to tell the stories of the doctors' paths from relative anonymity to becoming household names. I realize now that what I ended up with is also a book about journalism. In fact, its focus is a part of journalism I never thought much about until now: the essential role of the expert analyst, whose approach can guide—or in this case, elevate—the public's understanding of an important issue.

As you've read, their repeated appearances on air and in print took an extraordinary amount of their time. Not just the hours and hours on air, but also constantly keeping abreast of the data and theories. Sumon Chakrabarti talked about the "firehose" of information in first-year medical school. The flow of Covid data must have felt that way again during the early days of the pandemic.

The doctors' appearances also required a leap of faith. Faith that the media would treat them fairly. That we would give them time to make their points. That we would break out of the pattern of airing clips with opposing points of view that may seem like an exercise in balance: One expert says "A." The second says "B." The two points of view are played side by side with equal weight, and the audience is required to draw conclusions.

But with the pandemic, where our health depended on the decisions each of us made, we needed people who could assess the "A" and "B" and provide real-world answers when the real world was a scary place. Rather than an academic explanation of the data on fomite transmission of SARS-COV-2, we needed to know, in simple terms, what to do when we brought groceries into the house.

That is the void the infectious disease doctors stepped into. And while their profession is medicine, they took on their role as experts with an equal level of rigour. You could create a code of conduct for media experts based on how the doctors approached their interviews. No partisanship. No personal causes. Instead, a willingness to answer the questions we kept putting to them (even when, true story, it was a question from a viewer about whether flatulence could carry enough virus to infect someone else in a room).

There was a second leap of faith by these doctors: faith that the public would understand that the guidance they provided—even when it was based on careful analysis of the best science at the time—might change. Not because the answer was mistaken or the expert had "flip-flopped," but because this was science in real time, sometimes changing at hyper-speed.

And faith that the audience, including members of the scientific community, would realize that "Doc Talk"—those ubiquitous unscripted conversations with an informality that helped convey the message—might occasionally contain a verbal slip or a sentence made a little too dense by the artificial time constraints imposed by the media.

Most of our audience accepted that. But yes, we did get some feedback, some powered by a level of anger—"DON'T BE STUPID!! IT'S TAIWAN, NOT THAILAND"—that surprised me.

If they hadn't known it already, the doctors learned one of the biggest risks in fulfilling their duty: exposing themselves to criticism that often, especially when driven by social media, was very personal, fuelled by outrage and visible to everyone.

Perhaps because of their experiences dealing with patients, they had an impressive ability to distinguish between what might be truly dangerous and what was "merely" disturbing. But the reaction that seemed more discouraging to them was when some other scientists (including fellow physicians) turned nasty.

A few of the doctors told me that colleagues would sometimes question why they were appearing so often in the media, suggesting ego might be driving them. I have seen this in other professions, where an unwritten but iron-clad code of silence prevents the public from getting an informed, experienced perspective on an important issue.

With Covid, there was an additional and more corrosive peer pressure: criticism that undermined expertise. As one of the doctors told me, deep divides have opened up between some colleagues that will take a long time to repair. "This pandemic will come to an end, and there are people who will not be welcomed back. It's terrible to watch."

Faced with this kind of backlash, it would have been easy for the doctors profiled in this book to disappear behind the walls of their hospitals. But not once did I see those pressures prevent them from saying, in public, what they knew was right.

In the opening chapter I mentioned that if they were in the United States, some would probably have been offered their own television show by now. Looking back, I'm glad that didn't happen (or at least hasn't happened yet). While they did have ways to get their message directly to the public— social media and, to an extent, newspaper commentaries—I think we were better served by having their messages delivered on TV or radio news programs.

You might be thinking this comment is self-serving, coming from a journalist. A lot of people regard the "media filter" as a bad thing, with journalists using their lens to distort the message. But when it's done right, that media lens focuses on what's important and magnifies what's credible and clear. Each media organization was able to look through the many statements from many people and offer up our version of what we thought was credible and important.

In the end, it's not a coincidence that various outlets tended to rely on the same doctors. I've mentioned before that this is a very competitive business. We are always looking for new angles, exclusive information, experts no one else is using. To the credit of the infectious disease docs, they answered everyone's call. I wish we at the CBC had them all to ourselves, but, in keeping with their sense of duty, that was never an option.

Not being offered their own afternoon talk show highlights a very Canadian phenomenon. Even when telegenic doctors become household names, rather than promoting their own line of immune-boosting vitamins on daytime television, they keep doing interviews on their laptop from their home office, for free (and, for the record, none of them have a line of vitamins).

And that brings me back to something I wrote about earlier: what this group says about our country. They are a portrait of successful, hard-working Canada, almost equally divided between men and women, with diverse backgrounds. Coming here from many countries, their families were part of a scientific diaspora that produced, among other things, a lot of doctors.

Another point worth repeating is how many of them went to their hometown university. I think it's something about Canada we don't fully appreciate. We don't have a small number of elite schools where you need to go for your undergraduate studies if you want to be, or are perceived to be, ambitious and successful.

These doctors also showed you don't have to have a single-minded focus on medicine from high school to under-grad to first-year med school—with the obvious exception of five-year-old Sumon! Think about Lynora Saxinger considering medical school on a whim—"I'm smarter than that guy, he's applying to medicine, should I apply to medicine?"; Fatima Kakkar doing her undergraduate studies in political science—"they're very different than the science crowd"; or Isaac Bogoch, on a Brisbane beach, wondering if he should try to defer his medical school acceptance for another year—"I was having the time of my life."

Let me finish with one more thank-you to all nine of these doctors, for all that they were willing to do during this pandemic, but also for their candour in talking to me for this book. That took some faith as well, in how I would tell their stories but also how you would read them.

I'm glad they got to enjoy some of the benefits of their public profile and were willing to share the surprises (some patients paying more attention to their advice), the fun (like Murthy's "Most Likely to Save the World" award from his high school's grad class) and the gratifying moments (so many people, some asking for physically distanced selfies, thanking the doctors for their service).

Who doesn't like a little public adulation for doing their duty? But I'll give Sumon Chakrabarti the last word, versions of which I heard from every single doctor: "Being recognized, understood that what I'm trying to do is help, that's been a good thing. But when this is all over, I'll be quite happy to return to anonymity."

If that is a sign the pandemic is over, I think we'll all be happy to see them return to anonymity. But I'll miss them.

ACKNOWLEDGMENTS

To THE DOCTORS. I ASKED FOR TWO FORTY-FIVE-MINUTE phone conversations. Without hesitation you provided more.

To the "talk team" producers at *The National*. I can't even guess how many hours you spent on Covid interviews.

And to the editor, Audrey McClellan. I am so impressed by your ability to suggest changes—LOTS of little changes—that retained my voice but made this book so much better.

INDEX